Anesthesia and Co-Existing Disease

Edited by

ROBERT N. SLADEN, MD

Professor and Vice-Chair
Department of Anesthesiology
Chief, Division of Critical Care
Director, Cardiothoracic and Surgical Intensive Care Units
Columbia University
College of Physicians and Surgeons
New York, NY

DOUGLAS B. COURSIN, MD

Professor
Departments of Anesthesiology and Internal Medicine
University of Wisconsin Medical School
Madison, WI

JONATHAN T. KETZLER, MD

Associate Professor
Departments of Anesthesiology and Critical Care Services
University of Wisconsin Medical School
Madison, WI

HUGH PLAYFORD, MD

Assistant Professor
Department of Anesthesiology
Associate Program Director
Critical Care Fellowship
Columbia University
College of Physicians and Surgeons
New York, NY

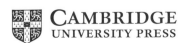

CAMBRIDGE
UNIVERSITY PRESS

CAMBRIDGE UNIVERSITY PRESS

Cambridge, New York, Melbourne, Madrid, Cape Town, Singapore, São Paulo, Delhi

Cambridge University Press

32 Avenue of the Americas, New York, NY 10013-2473, USA

www.cambridge.org

Information on this title: www.cambridge.org/9780521709385

First published 2007

Printed in the United States of America

A catalog record for this publication is available from the British Library

**WO
200
A5775
2007**

Library of Congress Cataloging in Publication Data

Anesthesia and co-existing disease / Robert N. Sladen ... [et al.].
    p. ; cm.
ISBN-13: 978-0-521-70938-5 (pbk.)
ISBN-10: 0-521-70938-5 (pbk.)
1. Anesthesia.   2. Anesthetics – Side effects.   I. Sladen, Robert N.
[DNLM: 1. Anesthesia – methods.   2. Anesthesia – adverse effects.
3. Perioperative Care – methods. WO 200 A5775 2007]
RD82.A6594   2007
617.9′6–dc22   2007016739

ISBN   978-0-521-70938-5 paperback

Every effort has been made in preparing this book to provide accurate and
up-to-date information that is in accord with accepted standards and practice at
the time of publication. Nevertheless, the authors, editors, and publisher can make
no warranties that the information contained herein is totally free from error, not
least because clinical standards are constantly changing through research and
regulation. The authors, editors, and publisher therefore disclaim all liability for
direct or consequential damages resulting from the use of material contained in
this book. Readers are strongly advised to pay careful attention to information
provided by the manufacturer of any drugs or equipment that they plan to use.

NOTICE

Because of the dynamic nature of medical practice and drug selection and dosage, users are advised that decisions regarding drug therapy must be based on the independent judgment of the clinician, changing information about a drug (e.g., as reflected in the literature and manufacturer's most current product information), and changing medical practices.

While great care has been taken to ensure the accuracy of the information presented, users are advised that the authors, editors, contributors, and publisher make no warranty, express or implied, with respect to, and are not responsible for, the currency, completeness, or accuracy of the information contained in this publication, nor for any errors, omissions, or the application of this information, nor for any consequences arising therefrom. Users are encouraged to confirm the information contained herein with other sources deemed authoritative. Ultimately, it is the responsibility of the treating physician, relying on experience and knowledge of the patient, to determine dosages and the best treatment for the patient. Therefore, the author(s), editors, contributors, and the publisher make no warranty, express or implied, and shall have no liability to any person or entity with regard to claims, loss, or damage caused, or alleged to be caused, directly or indirectly, by the use of information contained in this publication.

Further, the author(s), editors, contributors, and the publisher are not responsible for misuse of any of the information provided in this publication, for negligence by the user, or for any typographical errors.

Contents

PART TWO. PHARMACOLOGY

Preface

Anesthesia and Co-existing Disease provides a timely, rapid overview of common and uncommon co-morbidities that are encountered in the day-to-day practice of anesthesiology. It provides a guide to the perioperative assessment and anesthetic management of patients with widely prevalent co-morbidities such as hypertension, diabetes, obesity, myocardial ischemia, and kidney and liver disease. It concisely outlines priorities for patients with special problems who are undergoing unrelated operative procedures, such as the obstetrical patient, the patient with prior organ transplantation, the adult patient with congenital heart disease, the spinal cord injured patient, the cancer patient with prior chemotherapy, the critically ill patient, or the patient with a psychiatric disorder. It also focuses on specific challenges to the anesthesiologist, such as patients with latex allergy, a history of substance abuse, preoperative use of herbal medications, or those who are at risk of malignant hyperthermia.

This text consists of 57 individual chapters with a structured outline format that starts with a description of the disease or condition. Subsections address its impact on fluid and electrolyte management, the cardiopulmonary system, hematologic reserve, gastrointestinal function, metabolism and nutrition, neurologic and psychiatric function. Next, the pharmacologic implications – pharmacokinetic and pharmacodynamic – enumerated. In the third component, subsections tackle preoperative evaluation, risk stratification, and preparation; intraoperative priorities, preparation, monitoring, and care; and finally postoperative management, pain control, PACU issues, and intermediate care or ICU requirements and indications.

Anesthesia and Co-Existing Disease is not intended to be an exhaustive or referenced text. Instead, it is a uniquely portable hands-on guide that provides a logical approach to acute perioperative care for adult patients with common or specialized needs. This multi-authored resource draws from a host of experts in identifying important issues, establishing perioperative priorities, and providing management guidelines in a consistent and easily accessible format.

Robert N. Sladen
Douglas B. Coursin
Jonathan T. Ketzler
Hugh Playford

PART ONE

Disease

ADRENAL & PITUITARY DISEASE

GIUDITTA ANGELINI, MD

OVERVIEW

- Pituitary adenomas represent 10–15% of intracranial neoplasms.
- Prevalence is 200/1,000,000; post-mortem incidence is 10–27%.
- Significant number are asymptomatic.
- Most pituitary tumors arise from anterior lobe (adenohypophysis)
  - Majority are benign.
- 75% of tumors secrete hormones inappropriately
  - Prolactin
  - Growth hormone (GH): acromegaly
  - Premature puberty or resumption of menstrual bleeding in postmenopausal women
  - Adrenocorticotrophic hormone (ACTH): Cushing's syndrome
- Presentation variable
  - Hormonal hypersecretion syndrome (see above)
  - Mass effect (non-secreting macroadenomas >1 cm): visual disturbance (bitemporal hemianopsia/third nerve palsy) or increased ICP
  - Nonspecific symptoms, such as headache, infertility, pituitary hypofunction or epilepsy (compression from nonfunctioning adenoma, secondary hyperprolactinemia, apoplexy or infarction)
  - Incidental finding

FLUID & ELECTROLYTES

- Acromegaly
  - Diabetes

- Cushing's syndrome
  - Diabetes
  - Hypernatremia, hypokalemia & alkalosis
  - Renal calculi
- Hypopituitarism
  - Hyponatremia, hyperkalemia & acidosis

CARDIOPULMONARY
- Acromegaly
  - Hypertension
  - Cardiomegaly, impaired LV function (interstitial fibrosis)
  - Obstructive sleep apnea (OSA): macroglossia, thickened pharyngeal tissues
- Cushing's syndrome
  - Hypertension
  - ECG: LVH, high-voltage QRS, inverted T waves; reversible w/ pituitary removal

HEMATOLOGIC
N/A

METABOLIC-NUTRITIONAL
- 5 distinct cell types plus null (functionally inert) cells
  - 50% somatotrophs: secrete GH
  - 10–25% lactotrophs: secrete prolactin
  - 15% corticotrophs: secrete ACTH
  - 10% gonadotrophs: secrete follicle-stimulating hormone (FSH) & luteinizing hormone (LH)
  - 5–10% thyrotrophs: secrete thyroid-stimulating hormone
- Production & release of anterior pituitary (adenohypophysis) hormones under control of hypothalamus:
  - Prolactin stimulated by prolactin-releasing hormone (PRH) & inhibited by dopamine
  - GH stimulated by growth hormone-releasing hormone & inhibited by somatostatin

- ➤ Thyroid-stimulating hormone (TSH) stimulated by thyroid-releasing hormone (TRH)
- ➤ ACTH stimulated by corticotrophin-releasing hormone (CRH)
- Anterior pituitary hormones are under feedback control.
  - ➤ Insulin-like growth factor I directly inhibits GH but also stimulates secretion of somatostatin.
  - ➤ Thyroid hormones inhibit both TSH & TRH.
  - ➤ FSH & LH have both inhibitory & stimulatory effects on the pituitary & hypothalamus.
- Posterior (neurohypophysis) secretes oxytocin & arginine vasopressin (AVP).

GASTROINTESTINAL
- Cushing's syndrome is associated w/ gastroesophageal reflux disease (GERD).

NEUROPSYCHIATRIC
- Cushing's syndrome is associated w/ mental disturbance.

ADULT CONGENITAL HEART DISEASE

MARY E. McSWEENEY, MD

OVERVIEW
- Adults w/ CHD may remain undiagnosed until adulthood.
- Adults may have had 1 or more corrective or palliative cardiac procedures.
- Clinical picture: ranges from essentially normal physiology to critically ill
- End-stage adult CHD: severe pulmonary hypertension (PHT) & Eisenmenger physiology

Congenital defects fall into 3 groups:
- Shunt lesions resulting in increased pulmonary blood flow (PBF)

- Shunt lesions resulting in decreased PBF
- Obstructive lesions, resulting in increased cardiac work & impaired blood flow distal to the obstruction

Two major consequences of the abnormal anatomy:
- Cyanosis: decreased pulmonary artery (PA) blood flow or mixing of systemic & pulmonary venous (PV) return
- CHF: increased PA blood flow, from excessive PV return, or impaired PV return from obstruction or impaired forward cardiac output (CO). Both lead to pulmonary vascular congestion.

Classification of CHD also depends on surgical status:
- Anatomy may be unchanged or previously surgically altered by a corrective or palliative procedure.
- Surgical correction of complex lesions (eg, single ventricles) is often staged.
- Corrective procedures can themselves induce heart block or impair ventricular function.

Acyanotic lesions
- Ventricular septal defect (VSD)
  - Chronic volume overload results in abnormal ventricular function. Pts repaired after 5 yrs of age are likely to have residual ventricular dysfunction.
  - Nonrestrictive or moderately restrictive VSDs cause pulmonary vascular pressure/volume overload & PHT. Ultimately, reversal of shunt results in Eisenmenger physiology.
- Atrial septal defect (ASD)
  - Simple ostium secundum defect is the most common shunt lesion in adults.
  - May be asymptomatic & permit survival into late adulthood

➤ Most pts >60 yrs old are symptomatic: increased systemic arterial pressure & decreased ventricular compliance cause increased L-to-R shunt through the ASD.

➤ Atrial tachyarrhythmias are common > 40 yrs.

➤ PHT develops > 40 yrs.

➤ Pts w/ normal pulmonary pressures corrected surgically before 24 yrs have normal survival.

➤ Paradoxical emboli (from atrium to cerebral vessels) may occur because of preferential streaming of blood flow from IVC across foramen ovale (secundum ASD), especially during sudden increases in PVR (coughing, etc.).

■ Partial anomalous pulmonary venous connection

➤ Partial pulmonary venous return to right atrium (RA)

➤ Wide variety of anomalous pulmonary venous connections, usually w/ sinus venosus ASD

➤ Physiology & natural history similar to ASD for similar degree of L-to-R shunt

➤ SA node dysfunction possible if sinus venosus type

➤ Scimitar syndrome: anomalous connection of all right PV to IVC, associated w/ hypoplastic right lung (arterial circulation to right lung from descending thoracic aorta)

■ Coarctation of the aorta

➤ Commonly associated w/ bicuspid aortic valve

➤ Severe coarctation presents w/ heart failure within first wks of life.

➤ Milder coarctation: survive into adulthood

➤ Later repairs associated w/:
  • High incidence of hypertension in pts repaired late
  • Increased incidence of premature coronary artery disease

■ Pulmonary valve stenosis

➤ Most stenosis is noncritical; survival into adulthood is the rule.

- ➤ Associated w/ right ventricular (RV) hypertrophy & eventual RV failure
- ➤ Commonly repaired w/ balloon valvuloplasty
- ■ Congenitally corrected transposition of the great arteries (L-transposition, ventricular inversion)
  - ➤ Blood flow: RA → MV → LV → PA → lungs → LA → tricuspid valve → RV → aorta
  - ➤ Aorta located anterior & to the left of the main PA
  - ➤ Anatomic RV serves as systemic ventricle.
  - ➤ RV eventually vulnerable to failure
  - ➤ High incidence of heart block
- ■ Ebstein's anomaly of the tricuspid valve
  - ➤ Abnormal apical displacement of the tricuspid tissue → atrialized RV w/ tricuspid regurgitation
  - ➤ Sometimes w/ pulmonic stenosis

Cyanotic lesions

- ■ Tetralogy of Fallot (TOF)
  - ➤ Pulmonic stenosis, VSD, overriding aorta, RVH
  - ➤ Most common cyanotic lesion encountered in older pts
  - ➤ Uncorrected: 25% survival to adolescence; 3% >40 yrs
  - ➤ After early repair, LV ok, RV usually impaired
  - ➤ "Tet spell": increased R-to-L shunt secondary to decreased SVR; treated w/ phenylephrine to increase SVR (pulmonary resistance "fixed" from stenotic pulmonic valve)
  - ➤ "Tet spells" rare in older pts w/ uncorrected TOF
  - ➤ After repair, right bundle branch block (RBBB) common, sometimes associated w/ left anterior hemiblock
- ■ Palliated tetralogy of Fallot
  - ➤ Palliative shunts (Blalock-Taussig, Waterston-Cooley, Potts or Gore-Tex central aortopulmonary) to increase PBF
  - ➤ PBF dependent on relative PVR vs. SVR
- ■ Complete transposition of the great arteries (D-transposition)
  - ➤ Incompatible w/ life unless adequate mixing

- ➤ 4 types of repair
  - Mustard or Senning (atrial repair): systemic venous return → LV → PA & pulmonary venous return → RV → aorta
  - Arterial switch: aorta & coronary arteries transposed to arise from LV & PA moved to arise from RV; most common repair now
  - Rastelli: LV outflow channeled through the VSD to aorta & RV connected to PA by external conduit
  - Palliative atrial repair in presence of a VSD & pulmonic valve disease (least common)
- ➤ Post-repair physiology depends on repair type:
  - An RV that must function as a systemic ventricle is vulnerable to failure.
  - Atrial repair is associated w/ high incidence of electrophysiologic problems (SA node dysfunction, AV block, SVT, etc.).
- ■ Single ventricle physiology
  - ➤ Include those w/ tricuspid atresia or a single, double inlet ventricle, usually a morphologic left ventricle
  - ➤ Survival to adulthood depends on the anatomy: pulmonary stenosis (protects pulmonary vascular bed) & competent atrioventricular valve(s) increase survival.
  - ➤ Generally pts w/ single LV do better than pts w/ single RV (morphologic).
  - ➤ Pts w/ unrestricted PBF typically develop pulmonary vascular disease.
  - ➤ Pts w/ restricted PBF may have required palliative shunts to increase PBF (to treat hypoxia).
  - ➤ Aortopulmonary shunts result in volume overload of the single ventricle; over time this results in ventricular failure.
  - ➤ Cavopulmonary shunts (Glenn) increase PBF w/out volume overload of the single ventricle.

- Fontan procedure
  - ➤ RA to PA connection for "correction" of single-ventricle hearts
  - ➤ Two-stage procedure
  - ➤ Step 1: anastomosis of SVC to undivided right PA = bidirectional Glenn shunt
  - ➤ Step 2: IVC connected to PA via Gore-Tex graft through RA
  - ➤ Graft usually baffled into LA so that some R-to-L shunt persists as safety valve in cases of high pulmonary resistance
    - Fluid retention (effusions, ascites)
    - Forward flow depends on CVP exceeding LAP to provide driving force for PA blood flow.
    - Must have adequate intravascular volume & avoid increased PVR (see above)
- Truncus arteriosus
  - ➤ Truncus arteriosus w/ unobstructed PA origin from the ascending aorta rapidly results in fatal CHF w/out correction.
  - ➤ Survival is permitted by pulmonary vascular inflow stenosis/disease sufficient to limit L-to-R shunt (but cyanosis is increased).
  - ➤ Truncal valve often malformed & incompetent; regurgitation is biventricular & can be severe
  - ➤ Adult survivors: repair by closure of VSD & interposition of valved conduit between RV & PA
    - The truncal valve remains as the aortic valve & incompetence should be treated like aortic insufficiency.
    - The valved RV to PA conduit is prone to stenosis & insufficiency RV failure.
    - The conduit lies just beneath the sternum & is vulnerable to sternotomy.
- Total anomalous pulmonary venous connection
  - ➤ Obligatory R-to-L shunt resulting from pulmonary veins emptying into RA

➤ Pts w/ supradiaphragmatic PV connection, low PVR & a large ASD have natural history similar to that of isolated nonrestrictive ASD but w/ systemic arterial saturations in the low 90s.

■ Eisenmenger physiology/pulmonary vascular disease

➤ PVR at or above SVR w/ resultant R-to-L shunt

➤ Anatomy: nonrestrictive communications at great arterial, ventricular or atrial level, by heart w/ single ventricle or two ventricles w/ or w/out ventricular inversion

➤ Excessive PBF & pressure result in changes in PA vasculature & ultimately fixed high PVR.

➤ Confers high perioperative risk:

- Represents most of unoperated adults w/ CHD who are referred for preop anesthetic evaluation
- Fixed PVR precludes rapid adaptation to intraoperative hemodynamic changes.
- Variations in SVR produce changes in the magnitude of R-to-L shunting (decreased SVR leads to increased R-to-L shunt).
- Hypovolemia, hypotension, vasodilators & regional anesthesia are poorly tolerated & exacerbate R-to-L shunt.
- Distorted cardiac anatomy & R-to-L shunt obviate PA catheters (hazardous placement, inaccurate CO). Relative resistance of PVR vs. SVR can be monitored by changes in systemic arterial pulse oximetry (SpO_2).
- Fixed high PVR is unresponsive to pharmacologic treatment but exacerbated by cold, acidosis, hypercarbia, hypoxia, endogenous or exogenous catecholamines w/ alpha-adrenergic effects.

■ Aortopulmonary shunts

➤ Used in any defect associated w/ low PBF

➤ May be palliative until reparative procedure or definitive procedure can be done

- ➤ Ventricular function determined by cardiac abnormality & amount of volume overload produced by shunt
- ➤ Systemic arterial oxygen saturation depends on PBF, which depends on maintenance of high SVR vs. PVR. R-to-L shunt is exacerbated by any fall in SVR or increase in PVR.
- ➤ Types
  - Blalock-Taussig (BT): subclavian artery to pulmonary artery; subclavian artery usually ligated for use
  - Potts: PA to aorta; higher pressure, higher flow than BT shunt, results in development of pulmonary vascular disease
  - Central: main PA to aorta; similar hemodynamically to Potts

FLUID & ELECTROLYTES
N/A

CARDIOPULMONARY
- ■ Shunt lesions: pts are dependent on relative PVR vs. SVR for direction of blood flow.
- ■ Pts w/ long-standing increased pressure and/or volume load to the pulmonary vasculature ultimately develop PHT. This can lead to R-to-L shunting in pts w/ previous L-to-R shunts.
- ■ Blood flow across the non-shunt lesion is dependent on ventricular pumping against high resistance. Myocardial depression may cause decompensation.
- ■ Lesions w/ increased PBF cause decreased pulmonary compliance, which increases the work of breathing.

HEMATOLOGIC

Polycythemia
- ■ Cyanotic lesions & attendant hypoxemia result in increased renal erythropoietin, high hematocrit & hyperviscosity (if Hct > 65%).

- Dehydration increases thrombotic risk (especially in upper lobes of lungs when PVR is elevated). A bleeding diathesis also exists, not reliably related to thrombocytopenia.
  - ➤ Artifactually elevated PT & PTT: erythrocytosis, less plasma in sample to interact w/ citrate in blood tubes.

METABOLIC/NUTRITIONAL
N/A

GASTROINTESTINAL
N/A

NEUROPSYCHIATRIC
- Paradoxical emboli to CNS are a risk in any pt w/ lesions w/ R-to-L shunt.
- Lower extremity or pelvic veins: source of thrombotic emboli
- Hospitalized pts are at risk for air or particle emboli entering from peripheral or central venous catheters.
- Prior surgical nerve injury can cause deficits in recurrent laryngeal, phrenic or sympathetic chain function.

ALCOHOL ABUSE

JONATHAN T. KETZLER, MD

OVERVIEW
- Lifetime prevalence of alcohol (ETOH) abuse: 14–36%
- Alcohol abuse is common in surgical & trauma pts.
- In one study, 43% of surgical pts who had ETOH levels checked were positive.
- ETOH abuse is more common in surgical population than general public.
- At-risk drinking: >16 standard drinks per wk for men & >10 drinks per wk for women

■ WHO defines "harmful drinking" as ETOH consumption that results in physical or psychological harm.

FLUID & ELECTROLYTES
■ May have very poor nutritional status

CARDIOPULMONARY
■ 3 possible mechanisms for myocardial damage
➤ An acute & transient toxic effect on cardiac performance, resulting in impaired myocardial contractility. This effect on myocardial function can become permanent w/ chronic alcohol consumption.
➤ Nutritional deficiency, particularly of thiamine, which can lead to beriberi heart disease
➤ Additives to an alcoholic beverage (eg, cobalt) may rarely exert a toxic effect on the myocardium.
■ The prevalence of alcoholic cardiomyopathy is similar in men & women w/ no significant differences in age or nutritional, clinical & radiologic parameters of heart failure.
■ Alcohol can produce asymptomatic cardiac dysfunction even when ingested by healthy individuals in smaller quantities, as during social drinking.
■ The risk of developing left ventricular dysfunction & alcoholic cardiomyopathy is related to both the mean daily alcohol intake & the duration of drinking.
■ Most pts in whom alcoholic cardiomyopathy develops have been drinking >80 g ethanol per day for >5 yrs.
■ The pt w/ alcoholic cardiomyopathy presents w/ symptoms & physical findings that are similar to those in pts w/ a dilated cardiomyopathy of any etiology.

HEMATOLOGIC
■ Macrocytosis w/ or w/out anemia, leukopenia and/or thrombocytopenia

- Mechanism unknown but may be related to utilization of folic acid, direct toxic effect on hematopoietic cells or abnormalities in membrane phospholipids
- With abstinence & reasonable diet, pt may have rebound thrombocytosis w/ platelet counts of >900,000/microliter at 1–2 wks. Return to normal levels at 7–10 days.

METABOLIC/NUTRITIONAL
N/A

GASTROINTESTINAL
- Prone to hepatic insufficiency w/ attendant esophageal varices
- Common to have chronic gastropathy
- Hepatic toxicity: acute alcoholic hepatitis, liver dysfunction, synthetic dysfunction, etc.
- Risk of pancreatitis

NEUROPSYCHIATRIC
- May have axonal degeneration of peripheral nerves
- CNS symptoms include memory loss, irritability & dementia.
- Withdrawal-associated seizures are generalized tonic-clonic & usually occur within 48 hrs of last drink.
- Usually single episodes & require no treatment
- 5% of pts who undergo withdrawal experience delirium tremens (DTs).
- DTs typically occur 48–96 hrs after last drink.
- Wernicke's encephalopathy secondary to thiamine deficiency
  - ➤ Cognitive dysfunction, especially memory disorders
  - ➤ Classic triad
    - Encephalopathy
      - Profound disorientation, indifference & inattentiveness
    - Oculomotor dysfunction

- Nystagmus, lateral rectus palsy & conjugate gaze palsies
  - Secondary to lesions of the oculomotor, abducens & vestibular nuclei
- Gait ataxia
  - Due to combination of polyneuropathy, cerebellar involvement & vestibular paresis
  - Wide-based gait w/ short steps

■ Korsakoff's amnestic syndrome is a late manifestation of Wernicke's.

ANEMIA

DOUGLAS B. COURSIN, MD, AND KARL WILLMANN, MD

OVERVIEW

■ Red blood cell (RBC) production normally matches red cell destruction.
  ➤ Normal life of an RBC is 110–120 days.
■ RBCs are generated in the bone marrow under the control of erythropoietin (EPO) & various cytokines.
  ➤ EPO is a trophic hormone produced in the macula densa of the kidney.
    - Modulated by the adequacy of tissue O_2 delivery
      - Therefore, it should increase w/ anemia, hypoxemia & decreased O_2 delivery to the kidney.
      - Various cytokines may alter normal EPO responsiveness.
        - May be cause of some anemias of chronic disease & ICU illnesses
■ Reticulocytes are young RBCs & normally represent 1.5% of circulating RBCs.
■ Reticulocyte count normally increases as response to anemia.

- Anemia is defined as a reduction below the normal limits of RBCs in the circulation.
  - ➤ Iron deficiency is most common nutrient deficiency.
  - ➤ Incidence of anemia increases w/ age.
  - ➤ About 2.5% of the population has a physiologic anemia.
- Determine etiology, degree of anemia, physiologic effect & need, if any, to treat immediately or treat during OR/ICU care.
  - ➤ Signs & symptoms of anemia depend on the degree of anemia, speed with which the anemia developed & individual physiologic reserve.
  - ➤ Symptoms are related to decreased O_2 delivery & if actively bleeding or inadequately compensated, degree of hypovolemia.
- Hemoglobin (Hgb): concentration of the oxygen-carrying pigment in whole blood
  - ➤ Normal Hgb for male: 15.7 +/− 1.7 mg/dL; anemic if Hgb < 13.5 mg/dL
  - ➤ Normal Hgb for female: 13.8 +/− 1.5; anemic if Hgb < 12 mg/dL
    - Pts living at altitude frequently have higher normal values secondary to hypoxia-induced increased erythropoiesis.
    - Smokers & those exposed to some environmental pollutants may have higher Hgb, which may approach polycythemic levels.
    - Some athletes may have higher baseline Hgb.
    - As pts age, some develop a physiologic anemia; however, need to rule out underlying pathology such as colon cancer, GI blood loss or other.
- Hematocrit (Hct) is the percent of a volume of whole blood that is occupied by intact RBCs.
- Red cell count: number of RBCs in a volume of whole blood, millions of RBCs/microliter

- When measuring Hgb, Hct & red cell volume, take into account clinical scenario, speed of onset of anemia, presence of bleeding & overall volume status.
- Most important physiologic effect of anemia is decrease in tissue oxygen delivery
  - Can compensate as long as there is adequate intravascular volume, good cardiac function, reflex production of 2,3-DPG & decreased blood viscosity
  - Hgb disassociation curve shifts to the right in anemia, which facilitates O_2 release & delivery.

FLUID AND ELECTROLYTES

- RBCs circulate in plasma, which is essentially a non-cellular balanced salt solution w/ plasma proteins & coagulation factors.
- Exogenous RBCs should be administered in normal saline-based solutions to avoid hemolysis, crenation or chelation of preservative-based anticoagulants.

CARDIOPULMONARY

- Primary effect on cardiovascular system depends on whether anemia is normovolemic (well tolerated) or hypovolemic (poorly tolerated).
- Effects depend on rapidity & severity of anemia & pt reserve.
- Acute anemia has high potential for inducing myocardial ischemia in susceptible pts.
- Chronic anemia may induce a nutritional cardiomyopathy: transfusion may not improve cardiac function but simply induce CHF & pulmonary congestion.

HEMATOLOGIC

- Etiology of anemia
  - Morphology (based on CBC-based indices or red cell size)
    - Microcytic: low MCV, MCHC, RBC index

- Iron deficiency anemia, sickle cell anemia, thalassemia, others
- Macrocytic: high MCV
  - Vitamin B_{12} or folate deficiency
- Mixed: combination of micro & macrocytic anemia
- Normocytic: anemia of chronic disease
- Mechanism (applied below)
  - Blood loss
    - Most commonly encountered etiology
    - May be obvious during surgery, trauma
    - Occult: GI, GU, retroperitoneal, internal, soft tissue, etc.
  - Iatrogenic
    - Excessive phlebotomy
  - Decreased RBC production
    - Nutrient-mediated
      - Iron deficiency
      - B_{12} deficiency (pernicious anemia)
        - Associated w/ degeneration of lateral & posterior white columns of spinal cord
        - Paresthesias, loss of proprioception & vibratory sense
        - Associated w/ hypothyroidism
      - Folate deficiency
        - Most common in alcoholic & postpartum pts
    - Bone marrow compromise
      - Aplastic anemia: absolute failure of marrow to make red cells
      - Marrow replacement w/ tumor, infection, other
      - Marrow fibrosis such as myelodysplasia
      - Drug- or irradiation-induced suppression
    - Hormonal deficiency
      - Erythropoietin (EPO)
        - Acute or chronic renal impairment

- Anemia of chronic disease
- Anemia of critical illness
- Rarely, autonomic dysfunction syndromes
  - Hypothyroidism
  - Androgen deficiency
- RBC destruction
  - Abnormal RBCs
  - Hemolytic anemia
    - Occurs when RBCs live <100 days
    - May be antibody-mediated
    - Inherited
      - Sickle cell anemia
      - Thalassemia
      - Spherocytosis
    - Acquired
      - Coombs-positive, drug-induced hemolysis
      - Thrombotic thrombocytopenic purpura (TTP)
      - Hemolytic-uremic syndrome (HUS)

METABOLIC-NUTRITIONAL
- See "Nutrient-Induced Anemia" under "Hematologic" section.

GASTROINTESTINAL
- GI losses are a common cause of occult anemia.
- Upper or lower GI blood loss
  - Upper
    - Drug-related: NSAIDs, ASA
    - ETOH-induced
      - Gastritis
      - Gastric ulcer
      - Varices
    - Peptic ulcer disease
    - Tumor

- Vascular
- Other
➣ Lower
  - Diverticula
  - Vascular
  - Tumor
  - Infectious
  - Other

Renal

- EPO secreted by kidney is responsible for RBC production in the marrow.
- Normally make more RBC precursors than needed, so pro-erythrocytes are recycled.
- EPO stimulation, say from anemia or hypoxemia, stimulates normal maturation of RBCs as well as increased production.
- Pts w/ acute or chronic renal failure are usually anemic & treated w/ EPO.
  - ➣ Subcutaneous or IV treatment, usually 3x weekly
  - ➣ Avoid excessive administration.
  - ➣ Side effects: seizures, DVT, stroke, hypertension

NEUROPSYCHIATRIC

- Pts w/ pernicious anemia may have symptoms from vitamin B12 deficiency.

ANKYLOSING SPONDYLITIS

HUGH R. PLAYFORD, MD

OVERVIEW
N/A

FLUIDS AND ELECTROLYTES
N/A

CARDIOPULMONARY

- TMJ arthritis
- Cricoarytenoid arthritis
- Pleuritic inflammation
- Chest rigidity w/ restrictive pulmonary disease
  - ➤ Compensation by increased diaphragmatic contribution, thorax fixed at higher lung volumes, chest wall symmetry retained
- Upper lobe cavitation (rare)
- Cardiomyopathy
- Conduction defects
- Aortitis & aortic insufficiency

HEMATOLOGIC

N/A

METABOLIC-NUTRITIONAL

N/A

GASTROINTESTINAL

- Irritable bowel syndrome

NEUROPSYCHIATRIC

- Radiculopathy
- Atlantoaxial subluxation
- Vertebrobasilar insufficiency
- Occult spinal fracture
- Sacroiliitis
- Joint ankylosis
- "Bamboo spine"
- Spondylodiscitis
- Chronic back pain
- Cauda equina syndrome (rare)

ANTICOAGULATION THERAPY

JONATHAN T. KETZLER, MD

OVERVIEW

- In April 2002 the American Society of Regional Anesthesia & Pain Medicine convened its Second Consensus Conference on Neuraxial Anesthesia & Anticoagulation.
- Although the statements are based on a thorough evaluation of the evidence, data are sparse.
- The final decision about the use of regional anesthesia in anticoagulated pts is left to the judgment of the responsible anesthesiologist.
- The consensus focuses on neuraxial blocks, leaving the risk of plexus & peripheral blocks undefined.

FLUID AND ELECTROLYTES
N/A

CARDIOPULMONARY
N/A

HEMATOLOGIC
N/A

METABOLIC/NUTRITIONAL
N/A

GASTROINTESTINAL
N/A

NEUROPSYCHIATRIC
N/A

AORTIC REGURGITATION

ROBERT N. SLADEN, MD

OVERVIEW
- Etiology
  - Rheumatic fever
  - Congenital disease (Marfan's syndrome, Ehler-Danlos syndrome, etc.)
  - Acquired disease (syphilis, aortic dissection)
- Variable onset, slow progression, manifests in third to sixth decade
- Cardinal
  - Dyspnea
  - Syncope
  - Congestive heart failure

FLUID/ELECTROLYTE
N/A

CARDIOPULMONARY
- Hemodynamic profile: hyperdynamic
- Left ventricle (LV) undergoes eccentric hypertrophy & dilation (volume overload)
  - EF is increased > 0.6 while compensated
  - Restricted forward cardiac output: impaired circulatory reserve, effort intolerance, dyspnea
- Diagnosis
  - Wide pulse pressure ("water hammer" or "collapsing" pulse)
  - Harsh systolic + early diastolic murmur ("to & fro") at left sternal border
  - Cardiomegaly on chest x-ray
  - Left ventricular hypertrophy (LVH) on ECG
  - Increasing aortic regurgitation (TTE, TEE)

- Acute decompensation (low cardiac output syndrome)
  - Acute atrial fibrillation, tachyarrhythmias (loss of atrial kick)
- Late manifestations
  - Congestive heart failure
  - Sudden death
- Increased risk of perioperative myocardial ischemia
  - Very low diastolic perfusion pressure (may be close to 0)
  - Increased cardiac output requires increased heart rate (fixed stroke volume).

HEMATOLOGIC
N/A

METABOLIC/NUTRITIONAL
N/A

GASTROINTESTINAL
N/A

NEUROPSYCHIATRIC
N/A

AORTIC STENOSIS

ROBERT N. SLADEN, MD

OVERVIEW
- Etiology
  - Rheumatic fever (rarely)
  - Bicuspid aortic valve
  - Calcific aortic sclerosis
- Variable onset, slow progression, manifests in third to sixth decade

- Cardinal symptoms & life expectancy after onset (w/out treatment)
  - Angina (3 yrs)
  - Syncope (2 yrs)
  - Congestive heart failure (1 yr)

FLUID & ELECTROLYTES
N/A

CARDIOPULMONARY
- Hemodynamic profile: hypodynamic
- Left ventricle (LV) undergoes concentric hypertrophy (pressure overload)
  - Ejection fraction (EF) is increased >0.7 (end-systolic collapse).
  - Restricted forward cardiac output: impaired circulatory reserve, effort intolerance, dyspnea
  - Syncope or sudden death may occur w/ LV outflow tract (LVOT) obstruction.
- Impaired myocardial oxygen balance (MVO_2)
  - Increased demand (increased afterload, contractility)
  - Decreased supply (decreased aortic diastolic pressure, thickened myocardium)
  - Angina may occur w/out coronary artery disease (CAD).
  - Earlier-onset angina w/ concomitant CAD
- Diagnosis
  - Narrow pulse pressure
  - Harsh "diamond-shaped" systolic murmur radiating to neck
  - Cardiomegaly on chest x-ray
  - Left ventricular hypertrophy (LVH) on ECG
  - Increasing gradient across aortic valve (critical: peak > 70 mm Hg, mean > 50 mm Hg)
  - Decreasing aortic valve area (normal, 2–4 cm^2, critical < 1.0 cm^2)

- Acute decompensation (low cardiac output syndrome)
  - Acute atrial fibrillation, tachyarrhythmias (loss of atrial kick)
  - Late manifestations
  - Congestive heart failure
  - Sudden death
- Increased risk of perioperative myocardial ischemia
  - Acute ischemia w/ relatively mild perturbations
  - Low cardiac output syndrome (unable to respond to postop demands)
  - Cardiac arrest: CPR may be unsuccessful in overcoming LVOT obstruction

HEMATOLOGIC
N/A

METABOLIC/NUTRITIONAL
N/A

GASTROINTESTINAL
N/A

NEUROPSYCHIATRIC
N/A

BRONCHOSPASTIC DISEASE

HUGH PLAYFORD, MD

OVERVIEW
N/A

FLUIDS AND ELECTROLYTES
- Usually normal
- Chronic systemic steroid use may lead to fluid retention, hypernatremia, hypokalemia.

- Severe asthma
  - ➤ May be dehydrated (high insensible respiratory loss w/ hyperventilation, poor intake)
  - ➤ Hypokalemia related to beta-2 agonists

CARDIOPULMONARY
- Typically related to:
  - ➤ Bronchospasm of bronchial smooth muscle
  - ➤ Mucus hypersecretion
  - ➤ Airway inflammation
- Symptoms & signs
  - ➤ May have no symptoms or signs during periods of normal to near-normal pulmonary function
  - ➤ Wheezing: turbulent gas flow during expiration. Absence of wheeze in severe acute asthma may reflect absence of airflow.
  - ➤ Cough: may range from nonproductive to copious tenacious mucoid sputum
  - ➤ Dyspnea often parallels the severity of the expiratory airflow obstruction & may be associated w/ tachypnea & hyperventilation.
  - ➤ Chest discomfort frequent
- Investigations
  - ➤ FEV1 & maximal mid-expiratory flow rate reflect the severity of the expiratory airflow obstruction.
  - ➤ Pts often present to hospital w/ FEV1 <35% of normal, or maximal mid-expiratory flow rate <20% of normal. When FEV1 returns to about 50%, symptoms decrease markedly.
  - ➤ Flow-volume loop: downward scooping of the expiratory limb of the loop
  - ➤ Between asthma attacks, FRC may be increased by 1–2 L, but TLC remains normal.
  - ➤ DLCO usually unchanged
  - ➤ ABG (between attacks): often normal

- ➤ ABG (mild asthma attacks): decreased $PaCO_2$ & respiratory alkalosis
- ➤ ABG (worsening airflow limitation): decreased PaO_2 (from increasing ventilation-perfusion mismatch) & increased $PaCO_2$ (fatigue w/ increased work of breathing)
- ➤ Chest x-ray: important in excluding other causes of respiratory failure; often normal but may have hyper-inflation
- ➤ ECG: may have right axis deviation & ventricular irritability (beta-2 agonists, acidemia)
- ■ Related to therapy
  - ➤ Beta-2 agonists: sympathetic stimulation, tachycardia, cardiac dysrhythmias
  - ➤ Methylxanthines (eg, theophylline): cardiac dysrhythmias

HEMATOLOGIC
- ■ Usually normal
- ■ May be associated w/ an eosinophilia
  - ➤ Eosinophilia may parallel the degree of airway inflammation & airway hyperreactivity.

METABOLIC-NUTRITIONAL
- ■ Usually normal
- ■ May have chronic changes related to long-term systemic steroid use

GASTROINTESTINAL
- ■ Usually normal
- ■ May have chronic changes related to long-term systemic steroid use (gastritis, peptic ulcer disease)

NEUROPSYCHIATRIC
- ■ Usually normal

- In severe acute asthma
  - ➤ Generalized myopathy may be present (related to beta agonists, steroids, non-depolarizing neuromuscular blockers)
  - ➤ Anxiety common (beta agonists, hypoxemia, dyspnea)

CARCINOID SYNDROME

GIUDITTA ANGELINI, MD

OVERVIEW

- Incidence 1–2/100,000 in North America
- Most commonly seen in fourth or fifth decade of life
- At diagnosis of carcinoid tumors, 10–20% of pts are found to have noncarcinoid malignancies.
- 10% have MEN-I
  - ➤ Evaluate for pancreatic, pituitary & parathyroid disease.
- Most common presentation w/out syndrome is GI bleeding, intestinal obstruction or appendicitis.
- Mostly GI & lung but can also be found in breasts & ovaries
- Metastases usually from tumors >2 cm in diameter
- 35% of pts w/ metastases have symptoms of syndrome; only 2–5% w/out metastases have syndrome.
- Histamine, serotonin & bradykinin are main hormones involved, but also kallikrein, substance P, prostaglandins, gastrin, corticotropin, neuron-specific enolase

FLUID AND ELECTROLYTES

- Hypoalbuminemia
- Hyperglycemia

CARDIOPULMONARY

- 20% of tumors occur in lung.
- Histamine

- ➤ Vasodilation
- ➤ Extravascular smooth muscle contraction
- Serotonin
  - ➤ Vasodilation
- Bradykinin
  - ➤ Vasodilation
  - ➤ Histamine release
  - ➤ Bronchoconstriction
- Hypertension, hypotension, bronchospasm are all symptoms of carcinoid syndrome.
- One third of pts w/ carcinoid syndrome have cardiac disease
  - ➤ Right ventricular wall fibrinous plaques
  - ➤ Tricuspid regurgitation
  - ➤ Pulmonic stenosis

HEMATOLOGIC

- Nonmetastatic tumors secrete hormones that reach the liver by the portal vein & are usually inactivated.
- Cutaneous erythematous flushing is characteristic of carcinoid syndrome.

METABOLIC-NUTRITIONAL

- Tryptophan depletion is associated w/ serotonin release.
- Pellagra can result from carcinoid syndrome.

GASTROINTESTINAL

- Most tumors are GI
  - ➤ 50% appendix
  - ➤ 25% ileum (usually source of metastases)
  - ➤ 20% rectum
- Liver metastases have direct access to systemic circulation to release hormones & produce syndrome.
- Serotonin causes increased motility.
- Abdominal pain, vomiting, diarrhea & hepatomegaly are all symptoms of carcinoid syndrome.

NEUROPSYCHIATRIC

N/A

CHEMOTHERAPEUTIC AGENTS

JONATHAN T. KETZLER, MD

OVERVIEW

■ Various combinations of chemotherapeutic agents are used to treat neoplasms.

■ Anesthesiologists must deal with pts whose organ systems have been impaired.

■ Categories of chemotherapeutic agents
  ➤ Alkylating agents
    • Nitrogen mustard
    • Cyclophosphamide
  ➤ Antimetabolites
    • Methotrexate
  ➤ Vinca alkaloids
    • Vincristine
  ➤ Antibiotics
    • Anthracyclines: doxorubicin (Adriamycin), daunorubicin, others
    • Bleomycin
  ➤ Enzymes
    • Asparaginase
  ➤ Synthetics
    • Cisplatin
  ➤ Hormones
    • Corticosteroids

FLUIDS/ELECTROLYTES

N/A

CARDIOPULMONARY

■ Cardiac toxicity

➤ Shock
- Cardiogenic shock
  - Congestive heart failure
    - Anthracyclines; doxorubicin, daunorubicin, idarubicin, epirubicin, mitoxantrone
    - CHF that is refractory to cardiac glycosides is the hallmark.
    - Toxicity is related to cumulative dose; threat increases after cumulative dose reaches 400 mg/m^2.
    - Factors that exacerbate effects
      - Radiation to mediastinum
      - Exposure to cyclophosphamide, vincristine, fluorouracil or another anthracycline
      - Calcium channel blockers
    - Acute myocarditis uncommon
    - Early ST-segment & T-wave changes not significant
    - Discontinue anthracycline if left ventricular ejection fraction is <35% or absolute decrease of >10%.
  - Myocardial ischemia & necrosis
    - Cisplatin, vinblastine, vincristine
    - Cyclophosphamide
      - After high dose used for bone marrow transplant
      - ECG changes, heart failure & pericardial effusions can occur days to wks after dosing.
    - 5-Fluorouracil
      - May induce coronary artery spasm within minutes to hrs after dosing
  - Pericarditis
    - Anthracyclines (rare)
    - Radiation
      - Approx. 50% of cases of thoracic radiation
      - Typically occurs 6 months to 2 yrs after treatment
      - Can also cause cardiac ischemia, fibrosis & tamponade

- Cardiac dysrhythmias
  - Cyclophosphamide, 5-fluorouracil, ifosfamide, amsacrine, Taxol, doxorubicin, interleukin-2
- Distributive shock
  - Pancreatitis
    - L-asparaginase
    - Treat w/ glucocorticoids.
  - Addisonian crisis
    - Glucocorticoid withdrawal
  - Septic shock
    - Busulfan, carboplatin, carmustine (BCNU), cyclophosphamide, cytarabine, etoposide, fludarabine, idarubicin, ifosfamide, melphalan, mercaptopurine, methotrexate, mitomycin, procarbazine, thiotepa, topotecan, doxorubicin
    - Due to prolonged myelosuppression
  - Anaphylaxis
    - Carboplatin, cisplatin, cytarabine, etoposide, L-asparaginase, melphalan, methotrexate, mitomycin, pentostatin, procarbazine, teniposide
- Hypovolemic shock
  - Cyclophosphamide, ifosfamide
    - Hemorrhagic cystitis
- Pulmonary toxicity
  - Chronic pneumonitis, pulmonary fibrosis
    - Offending drugs
      - Azathioprine, bleomycin, busulfan, carmustine, chlorambucil, cyclophosphamide, melphalan, methotrexate, mitomycin C
    - Clinical findings
      - Bibasilar "Velcro-like" rales
      - Hypoxemia, respiratory alkalosis. Pulmonary function tests show restrictive process w/ decreased diffusion of CO.

- Chest x-ray: bibasilar reticulonodular infiltrates
- Lung biopsy: interstitial inflammation & thickening, cellular atypia, fibrosis
- Treatment
  - Stop offending drug.
  - Corticosteroids 1 mg/kg/day prednisone equivalent
  - Avoid excessive supplemental oxygen.
➤ Hypersensitivity pneumonitis
- Offending drugs
  - Bleomycin, methotrexate, procarbazine
- Clinical findings
  - Subacute onset of dyspnea
  - Nonproductive cough
  - Headache, chills, rash
  - Chest x-ray: diffuse interstitial infiltrates, often acinar pattern
  - Lung biopsy: interstitial eosinophilic infiltrates w/ histocytic cells
  - Treatment
➤ Acute respiratory distress syndrome
- Offending drugs
  - Cyclophosphamide, cytarabine, interleukin-2, methotrexate, mitomycin, teniposide, all trans-retinoic acids
- Clinical findings
  - Acute onset
  - Rales, respiratory failure
  - Pulmonary artery occlusion pressure not elevated
  - Chest x-ray: pulmonary edema due to increased capillary permeability
  - Lung biopsy: pulmonary edema, focal hemorrhage & thrombi & hyaline membranes
- Treatment
  - Supportive

- High-dose corticosteroids in fibroproliferative phase controversial
- ➤ Acute chest syndrome
  - Offending drugs
    - Bleomycin, methotrexate
  - Clinical findings
    - Pleuritic or retrosternal pain
    - Pleural rubs uncommon
    - Chest x-ray: normal
  - Treatment
    - Analgesia
- ➤ Bronchiolitis obliterans
  - Offending drugs
    - Bone marrow transplant
    - Occurs most commonly after lung transplantation
  - Clinical findings
    - Insidious onset cough & dyspnea on exertion w/ or w/out wheezing
    - Exam similar to emphysema
    - Pulmonary function tests: obstructive pattern
    - Chest x-ray: patchy infiltrates
    - Lung biopsy: lymphocytic or mixed inflammatory infiltrates w/ granulation tissue or fibrosis obstructing bronchiolar lumina
  - Treatment
    - Bronchodilators
    - High-dose corticosteroids
    - Immunosuppression controversial
- ➤ Radiation-induced pulmonary toxicity
  - Clinical findings
    - Dose-related toxicity
    - Dyspnea, cough, fever
    - Typically occurs 2–3 months after irradiation
  - Treatment

- Corticosteroids for acute toxicity but not recommended for fibrosis

HEMATOLOGIC
N/A

METABOLIC/NUTRITIONAL
N/A

GASTROINTESTINAL
- Nausea & vomiting
  - Offending drugs
    - Cisplatin, cyclophosphamide, cytarabine, hydroxyurea, doxorubicin, 5-fluorouracil, nitrosourea
- Mucositis
  - Offending drugs
    - Cytarabine, doxorubicin, 5-fluorouracil, hydroxyurea, methotrexate
  - Clinical findings
    - Grade 0: none
    - Grade 1: mild soreness, erythema, painless ulcers
    - Grade 2: painful erythema, edema or ulcers; able to eat
    - Grade 3: painful erythema, edema or ulcers; unable to eat
    - Grade 4: requires enteral or parenteral nutritional support
  - Treatment
    - Mouth care
      - Chlorhexidine gluconate rinse to reduce microbial colonization
      - Dyclonine hydrochloride rinse for topical analgesia
    - IV hydration
    - Sucralfate for cytoprotection
    - Nutritional support if necessary
- Diarrhea
  - Offending drugs

- Cytarabine, doxorubicin, 5-fluorouracil, hydroxyurea, methotrexate
- Veno-occlusive disease
  - Offending drugs
    - Mitomycin C, carmustine, busulfan, cyclophosphamide, dactinomycin, bone marrow transplant, radiation therapy
  - Clinical findings
    - Acute onset upper abdominal pain
    - Jaundice, hepatomegaly, ascites, oliguria
    - Hyperbilirubinemia, elevated serum transaminase activity
    - Hepatic biopsy: centrilobular cholestasis, hemorrhagic necrosis, central luminal obliteration
  - Treatment
    - Supportive therapy
    - 35% mortality in bone marrow transplantation
- Hepatotoxicity
  - Increased transaminase activity, alkaline phosphatase activity & bilirubin concentrations
    - Offending drugs
      - Cytarabine, hydroxyurea, L-asparaginase, 6-mercaptopurine, methotrexate, nitrosourea, pentostatin, plicamycin
  - Cirrhosis
    - Offending drugs
      - Methotrexate
  - Hepatic vein thrombosis
    - Offending drugs
      - Dacarbazine
  - Coagulopathy (decreased factors II, V, VII, X)
    - Offending drugs
      - L-asparaginase
  - Treatment
    - Supportive

NEUROPSYCHIATRIC
N/A

CHRONIC OBSTRUCTIVE PULMONARY DISEASE (COPD)

HUGH R. PLAYFORD, MBBS

OVERVIEW
N/A

FLUIDS & ELECTROLYTES
- May be mildly to moderately dehydrated by pt's high minute ventilation, diuretics
- Presence of hypokalemia may be related to beta-2-agonists and/or diuretics.

CARDIOPULMONARY
- Risk factors
  - ➤ External
    - Smoking (cigarette, cigar/pipe, passive), occupational exposure (miners, grain millers, etc.), environmental pollution
  - ➤ Internal
    - Genetic (alpha-1-antitrypsin deficiency), gender (male > female), socioeconomic status (poor), bronchial hyperresponsiveness, atopy & asthma, childhood illnesses (low birthweight, respiratory disease), dietary influences (vitamin C & E deficiency)
- Pathologic changes
  - ➤ Early stages: changes in large & small airways & lung parenchyma
  - ➤ Later stages: involvement of pulmonary circulation (medial hypertrophy of vascular smooth muscle & intimal hyperplasia, pulmonary hypertension), heart (right ventricular hypertrophy & failure, cor pulmonale) & respiratory muscles (atrophy)

- Clinically often separated as chronic bronchitis, emphysema
  - Chronic bronchitis
    - Mucus hypersecretion, decreased airway lumen due to mucus & inflammation, productive cough, normal diffusing capacity
    - Decreased FEV1, marked decrease PaO_2 ("blue bloater"), increased $PaCO_2$, DLCO normal, Hct increased, marked cor pulmonale
  - Emphysema
    - Destructive loss of lung parenchyma, loss of elastic recoil, possibly increased collagen deposition & fibrosis, airway collapse in exhalation, increased airway resistance, bullae formation w/ compression of adjacent lung tissue, increased work of breathing from reduced elastic recoil, decreased diffusing capacity, may be linked to alpha-1-antitrypsin deficiency (0.1% population, 5–10% of these also have hepatic disease)
    - Decreased FEV1, modest decrease PaO_2 ("pink puffer"), normal to decreased $PaCO_2$, decreased DLCO, normal Hct, mild cor pulmonale
- Physiologic changes
  - Permanent & minimally reversible obstruction to airflow during exhalation but w/ relatively preserved inspiratory flow
  - Characterized by progressive expiratory airflow limitation w/ FEV1 <65% predicted, FEV1/FVC <80%
  - Maximal inspiratory flow rate normal or near normal
  - Increased RV, increased FRC, increased work of breathing
- Symptoms & signs
  - Symptoms may not be present until relatively late; cough, dyspnea (often limiting exercise), ankle swelling, hepatic congestion
  - Slow & prolonged expiration, hyperinflation of thorax, distant breath sounds, may have wheeze, coarse early inspiratory crackles, use of accessory muscles of

respiration, signs of pulmonary hypertension, right heart enlargement and/or failure

➤ With extremis, asterixis & cyanosis

■ Investigations

➤ Chest x-ray: hyperlucency, hyperinflation, bullae

➤ ABGs: hypoxemia w/ advanced disease, hypercapnia & compensatory metabolic alkalosis w/ advanced disease

➤ PFTs: as above

➤ ECG: right heart strain (right axis deviation, RBBB, p pulmonale)

➤ Flow volume loops: early changes: scooped-out lower part of expiratory limb (abnormal flow at low lung volumes); later changes: scooping at all lung volumes

■ Implications

➤ High risk acute-on-chronic respiratory failure (upper & lower respiratory tract infections, surgery)

■ Therapies

➤ Bronchodilators (beta-2 agonists, hypokalemia, cardiac arrhythmias, tremor), mucolytics, anticholinergics (mild AE, dry mouth), steroids (inhaled & systemic, cataracts, osteoporosis, secondary infection, diabetes), methylxanthines (eg, theophylline, nausea/diarrhea/headache/seizures/cardiac arrhythmias), supplemental oxygen, intermittent antibiotics

HEMATOLOGIC

Polycythemia secondary to chronic hypoxemia

METABOLIC-NUTRITIONAL

■ High work of breathing increases metabolic load, elevated resting energy expenditure.

■ Malnutrition occurs in 25–33% of pts w/ moderate to severe COPD.

■ Depletion of fat mass & skeletal muscle mass

- Dyspnea, smoking may interfere w/ adequacy & style of nutrition.
- Significant deconditioning, particularly of respiratory muscles

GASTROINTESTINAL
Minimal change

NEUROPSYCHIATRIC
Minimal change

CHRONIC RENAL FAILURE

ROBERT N. SLADEN, MD

OVERVIEW
- Chronic renal disease
  - Chronic renal insufficiency (CRI)
  - End-stage renal disease (ESRD) (dialysis-dependent)
- Etiology
  - Primary (nephropathy)
  - Secondary (diabetes, hypertension, SLE, vasculitides)
- Dialysis
  - Hemodialysis (HD) (about 85% of pts)
  - Chronic ambulatory peritoneal dialysis (CAPD)

FLUID AND ELECTROLYTES
- Metabolic acidosis, hyperkalemia & congestive heart failure (CHF)
  - Well controlled by dialysis
- Anuric pts
  - Fluid loss is insensible only, about 500 mL/d.
- Polyuric chronic renal failure (CRF)
  - Urine output "normal", but concentrating ability absent
  - Fluid loss quickly results in hypovolemia.
- Moderate compensated anion gap acidosis

➤ Buffer base is depleted; bicarbonate (HCO_3-) 15–18 mEq/L
- Shock, diarrhea, hypercatabolism
  ➤ Rapid onset of metabolic acidosis
- Potassium (K), magnesium (Mg) & phosphate accumulate in CRF
  ➤ pH decrease of 0.1 can increase potassium by 0.5 mEq/L.
- Acute hyperkalemia
  ➤ Catabolic stress, acidosis
  ➤ K-sparing diuretics
  ➤ Red blood cell (RBC) transfusion
  ➤ K replacement
- Hyperkalemia
  ➤ Asystolic arrest (may occur w/out ECG prodrome)
- Hypermagnesemia
  ➤ Muscle weakness
  ➤ Increased susceptibility to muscle relaxants
- Hyperphosphatemia
  ➤ Renal osteodystrophy
- Excessive dialysis can result in K, Mg & phosphate depletion.
- Hypokalemia
  ➤ Supraventricular, ventricular arrhythmias
  ➤ Muscle weakness
- Hypomagnesemia
  ➤ Supraventricular, ventricular arrhythmias
- Hypophosphatemia
  ➤ Muscle weakness
  ➤ Increased susceptibility to muscle relaxants
  ➤ Difficult ventilatory weaning
  ➤ CNS dysfunction

CARDIOPULMONARY
- Pericarditis, hemorrhagic pericardial effusion
  ➤ Rare, well controlled by regular dialysis

- Systemic hypertension
  - Left ventricular hypertrophy (LVH) (may be asymmetric)
- Accelerated atherosclerosis, coronary artery disease (CAD)
  - Hypertension + hyperlipidemia + hyperglycemia
- Hyperdynamic circulation w/ fixed low systemic vascular resistance (SVR)
  - Anemia, arteriovenous shunts
  - Impaired circulatory reserve
  - Poor tolerance of myocardial ischemia or sepsis
- Increased risk of postop pulmonary edema, atelectasis & pneumonia
  - Hypoalbuminemia, low oncotic pressure, immune compromise
  - Abdominal distention (CAPD)

HEMATOLOGIC
- Normochromic, normocytic anemia (Hct 25–28%)
  - Decreased erythropoietin, red cell survival & chronic blood loss (GI tract, labs)
  - Increased cardiac output (CO)
  - Increased 2,3-diphosphoglycerate (2,3-DPG) (impaired by hypophosphatemia)
- Uremic coagulopathy (BUN > 60–80 mg/dL)
  - Defective endothelial release of von Willebrand's factor & factor VIII
  - Platelet function is abnormal.
  - Ivy bleeding time (BT) is prolonged >15 min (normal 3–8 min).

METABOLIC-NUTRITIONAL
- Disordered metabolism
  - Hyperglycemia (glucose intolerance)
  - Hypertriglyceridemia
  - Increased risk of atherosclerosis

- Protein malnutrition (kwashiorkor, hypoalbuminemic malnutrition)
  - Albuminuria
  - Dietary protein restriction
  - Losses via CAPD (10–40 g/d protein)
- Depleted lean body mass
  - Catabolic effects of uremia
  - Hypoalbuminemia, low colloid oncotic pressure (COP), interstitial & pulmonary edema
  - Decreased functional residual capacity (FRC), ventilatory reserve
  - Nosocomial & opportunistic infections (shunt or peritoneal catheter sites)
  - Wound dehiscence, fistulas, bedsores

GASTROINTESTINAL

- Anorexia, hiccups, nausea & vomiting (hallmarks of acute uremia)
  - Delayed gastric emptying
  - Increased risk of regurgitation & aspiration
- Mucosal inflammation, ulceration, bleeding (throughout GI tract)
- Peptic ulcer disease (25% of pts despite regular dialysis)
  - High incidence of hepatitis B and C
  - Anicteric carrier state in pts on chronic hemodialysis

NEUROPSYCHIATRIC

- Wide range of CNS manifestations
  - Subtle personality changes
  - Drowsiness, asterixis, myoclonus, seizures
- Acute encephalopathy
  - Major surgery, GI bleeding or infection
- Distal sensorimotor neuropathy
  - Concomitant autonomic neuropathy likely (see below)

> Important indication for dialysis
- Autonomic neuropathy
  > Delayed gastric emptying
  > Silent myocardial ischemia
  > Orthostatic hypotension
  > Impaired circulatory response to anesthesia

COCAINE TOXICITY

MARY E. McSWEENEY, MD

OVERVIEW

- Cocaine is the second most commonly used illegal drug in the US, after marijuana.
- Current users represent about 0.7% of the population; use is most common in males, age 18–25.
- Cocaine is an alkaloid made from the leaves of *Erythroxylon coca*, a shrub native to Central & South America, Indonesia & the West Indies.
- Cocaine is the only known naturally occurring local anesthetic.
- Consumption may be IV, intranasal or inhaled.
- First isolated in 1859, it was used in many products, including Coca-Cola, until banned in 1906 for nonprescription use.
- Most pts w/ a history of drug abuse deny it.
- Polysubstance abuse is common; consider toxicology screening.

FLUID AND ELECTROLYTES

- Rhabdomyolysis can lead to acute renal failure.

CARDIOPULMONARY

- Myocardial ischemia/infarction: acute coronary syndrome is the most common cardiac pathology associated w/ cocaine abuse. Up to 25% of nonfatal MIs in age group 18–45 are attributable to frequent cocaine abuse. Most MIs occur within 3 hrs of cocaine use, but this is variable. Anterior wall is the most frequent site of infarction. Pts often have normal coronaries. Ischemia mechanisms:

> Increased myocardial oxygen demand: sympathomimetic action increases myocardial inotropy, heart rate & systemic BP
> Coronary artery vasoconstriction/spasm: mediated by alpha-adrenergic receptors
> Coronary artery thrombosis: cocaine can activate platelets, increase platelet aggregability & potentiate thromboxane production

■ Arrhythmias & conduction abnormalities: arrhythmogenic potential is poorly understood: sinus tachycardia & bradycardia, bundle branch block, sudden death (ventricular fibrillation or asystole), ventricular tachycardia & accelerated idioventricular rhythm, heart block, torsades de pointes, a variety of supraventricular arrhythmias & an ECG pattern typical of Brugada syndrome (pseudo-right bundle branch block & persistent ST-segment elevation in V1-V3) have all been observed; arrhythmias disappear when drug is metabolized unless MI occurs

■ Myocarditis: mechanism unclear (infection, hypersensitivity reaction, etc.)

■ Cardiomyopathy: dilated cardiomyopathy secondary to unclear mechanism (direct toxic effect leading to destruction of myofibrils, interstitial fibrosis, myocardial dilation &heart failure suggested)

■ Acute aortic dissection

■ Left ventricular hypertrophy

■ Infective endocarditis (among IV users)

■ Pulmonary: pulmonary edema, infarction & hemoptysis, diffuse alveolar damage & bronchiolitis obliterans w/ organizing pneumonia (BOOP); crack cocaine is associated w/ "crack lung": diffuse alveolar infiltrates, eosinophilia & fever

HEMATOLOGIC
N/A

METABOLIC/NUTRITIONAL
N/A

GASTROINTESTINAL
- Mesenteric ischemia & infarction

NEUROPSYCHIATRIC
- Stroke: increased risk secondary to vasospasm, thrombus formation, vasculitis
- Combative behavior
- Altered pain perception

CONGESTIVE HEART FAILURE

MUHAMMED ITANI, MD, AND JONATHAN T. KETZLER, MD

OVERVIEW
- Affects 1% of adults in the USA
- Mortality rate is about 40% during first 4 years after diagnosis.
- Causes
  - Cardiac valvular abnormalities
  - Impaired myocardial contractility secondary to ischemia or cardiomyopathy
  - Systemic hypertension
  - Pulmonary hypertension

FLUIDS AND ELECTROLYTES
- Hyponatremia may occur.
- Hypokalemia is common in diuretic-treated pts.

- Salt restriction & diuretics often administered
- ACE inhibitors & aldosterone inhibitors such as spironolactone may induce hyperkalemia.

CARDIOPULMONARY
- Systolic dysfunction
  - ➤ Systolic wall motion abnormalities, localized w/ CAD, global w/ cardiomyopathy
  - ➤ Ventricular dysrhythmias common
  - ➤ Chronic hypertension produces pressure overload; valvular regurgitation may produce volume overload.
  - ➤ Hallmark: reduced LV EF (reflects severity of disease; measured w/ echocardiography, ventriculogram or radionuclide scanning)
  - ➤ LV dysfunction implies EF < 45% w/ or w/out symptoms
- Diastolic dysfunction
  - ➤ Age-dependent (<15% of pts <45 yrs, 35% of pts >65 yrs)
  - ➤ Hallmark: impaired ventricular relaxation
  - ➤ May have symptoms w/ normal systolic function
  - ➤ Higher filling pressures are required, which reflect back on the pulmonary system, causing pulmonary congestion & pulmonary edema depending on severity.
  - ➤ Most common causes: ischemic heart disease, aortic valve stenosis, chronic essential hypertension
  - ➤ Affects women > men
- Resting cardiac output may be normal but may not increase w/ exercise; eventually resting cardiac output becomes abnormal too (<2.5 L/min/m^2).
- Increased arteriovenous O_2 content difference due to increased O_2 extraction
- Pts may have concentric LV hypertrophy (w/ pressure overload) or eccentric LV hypertrophy (w/ volume overload); eventually LV will dilate & both systolic & diastolic dysfunction may coexist.

- Beta-receptor density is decreased in cardiac muscles in CHF & there is a decrease in response to beta agonists.
- Catecholamines are depleted in cardiac muscles & contractility is reduced.
- Stroke volume is relatively fixed; cardiac output can be increased only by increasing heart rate.
- Sympathetic nervous system overactivation causes arteriolar & venous constriction; therefore, BP is maintained & volume is shifted centrally toward the heart & brain.
- LV end-diastolic pressure (LVEDP) is elevated (normal: 12 mm Hg) due to increased LV stiffness & LV end-diastolic volume.
- LVEDP can be approximated from LA pressure in absence of mitral valve disease & from pulmonary artery diastolic pressure in absence of pulmonary artery disease.
- Increased LA pressure can be seen on EKG as P wave >0.1 sec & M-shaped configuration lead II
- Pulmonary edema is the ultimate manifestation of CHF.
  - ➤ Signs & symptoms: tachycardia, hypertension
  - ➤ PCWP > 30 mm Hg
  - ➤ Ratio of colloid osmotic pressure of edema fluid/plasma < 0.6

HEMATOLOGIC
- Anemia not uncommon in advanced CHF
- Correction of anemia associated w/ improved survival

METABOLIC-NUTRITIONAL
- Catecholamine depletion in the cardiac muscles w/ decreased contractility; urinary catecholamines are increased in CHF
- Renal blood flow is reduced, so renal tubular sodium & water retention increases to increase blood volume & maintain an adequate cardiac output; this can cause worsening of CHF & should be treated w/ vasodilators & ACE inhibitors. Prerenal azotemia is seen as BUN/CR > 20.

- Atrial natriuretic peptide production is reduced.
- Aldosterone release is suppressed & ADH release is increased.

GASTROINTESTINAL

- Liver congestion & enlargement w/ right heart failure
- Manifests as RUQ pain w/ rapid engorgement
- May have moderate to severe liver function test changes depending on severity
- Ascites: late finding, may happen secondary to liver dysfunction, constrictive pericarditis or tricuspid stenosis

NEUROPSYCHIATRIC

- Decreased cerebral blood flow w/ severe CHF leads to confusion & somnolence.
- In the setting of atrial fibrillation, LA clotting & cerebral embolization w/ ischemic stroke may occur.
- Overactivation of sympathetic nervous system to maintain systemic BP

COR PULMONALE AND RHF

MUHAMMED ITANI, MD, AND JONATHAN T. KETZLER, MD

OVERVIEW

- Cor pulmonale: right ventricular (RV) enlargement secondary to pulmonary hypertension
- Third most common cardiac disorder in persons >50 yrs
- Male:female = 5:1
- Exhibited in 10–30% of hospitalized pts w/ CHF
- COPD is the most common cause.
- COPD causes pulmonary capillary loss & arterial hypoxemia leading to pulmonary vasoconstriction. If hypoxemia is sustained, pulmonary medial hypertrophy occurs, leading to irreversible pulmonary hypertension.

- Systemic acidosis causes a synergistic effect w/ arterial hypoxemia on pulmonary vasoconstriction.
- Prognosis directly dependent on severity of pulmonary disease
- Other cause of right heart failure: primary pulmonary hypertension

FLUIDS AND ELECTROLYTES
- RV overload is usually treated w/ diuretics.
- Electrolyte disturbances may occur secondary to diuretic therapy.
- Avoid excessive fluid administration. If needed, measure RV pressures using central venous line.
- In case of biventricular failure, a PA catheter may be needed.
- With isolated RV failure, PCWP is usually in normal range.

CARDIOPULMONARY
- RV impairment may be acute (eg, pulmonary embolism) or progressive (eg, pulmonary hypertension w/ COPD).
- Criteria for pulmonary hypertension: mean PA pressure > 20 mm Hg (normal upper limit 16 mm Hg), w/ normal PCWP (normal upper limit 12 mm Hg)
- Severity of pulmonary hypertension indicated by gradient btwn pulmonary artery diastolic pressure & PCWP
- Signs & symptoms
- Loud P component of S2 & diastolic murmur due to pulmonary valve incompetence
- Prominent A wave of RA pressure wave
- Tricuspid regurgitation on Doppler echo
- Jugular venous distention in overt RV failure
- May have LV dysfunction due to concurrent CAD
- Mean PA pressure > 35 mm Hg is moderate pulmonary hypertension.
- RV failure in COPD is exacerbated by pulmonary infection.

- Treatment goal is to return PaO_2, $PaCO_2$ & pH toward normal. Cor pulmonale is more responsive to treatment w/ COPD & less responsive if the cause of pulmonary hypertension is irreversible vascular smooth muscle hypertrophy.

HEMATOLOGIC

- Erythrocytosis (secondary to chronic hypoxemia) increases blood viscosity.
- Erythrocytosis & thrombocytosis increase viscosity, potential for spontaneous clotting.
- Increased potential for spontaneous pulmonary thrombus formation & pulmonary embolism
- Diuretics may increase blood viscosity & worsen situation.
- Long-term anticoagulation essential w/ warfarin & similar meds, in addition to antiplatelet meds

METABOLIC-NUTRITIONAL

- COPD: Respiratory acidosis due to CO_2 retention
- COPD: Arterial hypoxemia due to pulmonary capillary destruction
- Diuretics may produce metabolic alkalosis & aggravate ventilatory insufficiency by decreasing the efficacy of CO_2 as a respiratory stimulant.
- Electrolyte disturbances (especially K^+) may occur due to diuretic therapy.
- 10% of pts w/ pulmonary hypertension (usually females) report symptoms of Raynaud's phenomenon.
- Low plasma proteins are seen in pts w/ liver failure.

GASTROINTESTINAL

- Congestive hepatopathy may develop due to elevated right-sided pressures.
- Portal hypertension may develop, leading to hypersplenism & thrombocytopenia.

- Esophageal varices & esophageal bleeding may develop as a consequence.
- Liver failure: ascites & increased risk of spontaneous bacterial peritonitis

NEUROPSYCHIATRIC
- Medullary respiratory center becomes less sensitive to CO_2 (increased levels required to maintain ventilatory drive).
- Hepatic encephalopathy (w/ liver failure)
- Spontaneous thrombosis may occur in small terminal vessels & induce multiple infarcts.

DIABETES MELLITUS AND DIABETIC EMERGENCIES

DOUGLAS B. COURSIN, MD

OVERVIEW
- Etiology
  - ➤ Disease of dysregulation of glucose metabolism related to insulin deficiency, resistance and/or abnormal gluconeo-genesis
- Most common endocrinopathy
- Type 1 DM affects 0.4% of population
  - ➤ Most often autoimmune
  - ➤ Usually develops in childhood or adolescence
  - ➤ May first present in diabetic ketoacidosis (DKA)
  - ➤ Absolute deficiency of insulin, therefore obligate need for insulin
- Type 2 DM affects 8–10% of population (25–35 million Americans)
  - ➤ Usually older, inactive & overweight
    - Increasingly developing in younger adults; some may be active & fit
    - Some appear to be genetically linked

➤ Produce insulin, so need for insulin supplementation is individualized
➤ May be treated w/ diet, oral hypoglycemic agents, insulin or any combination of these
  • Stress hormone response may necessitate first-time need for insulin.
➤ 1/3 to 1/2 of type 2 pts do not know they are diabetic at the time of surgery.
➤ Major acute diabetic-related complications
  • Hypoglycemia
  • Hyperglycemia
  • DKA
  • Nonketotic hyperosmolar state
➤ Major chronic diabetic-related complications
  • Vascular disease
    • Cerebrovascular
    • Coronary
    • Hypertension
    • Peripheral vascular
  • Cardiac compromise
  • Renal insufficiency/failure
  • Autonomic & peripheral neuropathy
  • Retinopathy
  • Connective tissue abnormalities
    • Stiff joint syndrome
  • Increased infectious risk

FLUID AND ELECTROLYTES
■ Risk for hypovolemia secondary to glucosuria
  ➤ Key is to reduce serum glucose to less than renal threshold for reabsorption (<180 mg/dL).
  ➤ Marked hypovolemia in pts w/ DKA (type 1 diabetics) or nonketotic hyperosmolar state (type 2 diabetics)

■ Infuse glucose judiciously to avoid hypoglycemia after insulin is administered & to avoid excessive hyperglycemia.

■ Type 1 DM obligate need for insulin
  ➤ Lack of insulin leads to hyperglycemia w/ dehydration.
  ➤ Conversion to lipid metabolism results in ketogenesis & ketoacidosis.
    • Metabolic acidosis results in movement of potassium out of cell to correct acidosis & serum hyperkalemia. However, total body potassium is low because of urinary losses.
  ➤ DKA frequently results in hypomagnesemia & hypophosphatemia.
  ➤ Pts may become significantly hypovolemic; volume resuscitation a key to initial treatment of DKA.

■ Various electrolyte abnormalities are common in diabetics. These are related to volume status, acid-base & metabolic derangements & baseline or evolving renal dysfunction. Since renal insufficiency is so common in diabetes, seek hyperkalemia.
  ➤ Magnesium wasting common in advanced diabetic nephropathy

CARDIOPULMONARY

■ Increased risk of coronary artery disease, hypertension, CHF, systolic & diastolic dysfunction
  ➤ Coronary disease is the most common cause of death in diabetics.
  ➤ Coronary disease may be asymptomatic because of autonomic neuropathy; therefore, "silent ischemia" is a risk.
  ➤ Use of ACE inhibitors may slow progression of cardiac & renal disease in diabetics; therefore, they are increasingly used chronically.

- Many advocate holding ACE inhibitors on the day of surgery because of concerns over hypotension that may be refractory to vasopressors such as ephedrine.

➤ Beta blockers are underused in high-risk diabetic pts, those with prior MI or known ischemia or those undergoing major surgeries such as vascular & thoracic procedures.

- Monitor for neuroglycopenic sequelae while on beta blockers.
- Contraindications are those that are common to non-diabetics.

➤ Diastolic dysfunction is usually treated with beta blocker, calcium channel blocker or ACE inhibitor.

HEMATOLOGIC

- Increased incidence of chronic anemia, especially renal insufficiency
- Chronic renal-insufficient diabetic at increased risk of coagulopathy & platelet dysfunction

METABOLIC-NUTRITIONAL

- Type 1 diabetics have an obligate need for insulin.
- Type 2 pts may or may not need insulin or insulin combined w/ oral agents.
- Type 2 pts who are controlled w/ diet or oral agents may require insulin intraoperatively or perioperatively because of stress hormone response & insulin resistance & excessive gluconeogenesis or withdrawal of oral agent control.
- Hemoglobin A-1-c allows a look back at how well controlled the diabetic has been over the past 6 or so wks.
- Diabetics are at increased risk for additional endocrine dysfunction.

GASTROINTESTINAL

- Progressive renal compromise develops commonly in type 1 and type 2 DM.
- Evaluate w/ urinalysis to identify proteinuria, the first sign of diabetic nephropathy & bacteria, since bacteruria may be asymptomatic.
  - ➤ Degree of albuminuria correlates w/ risk for cardiovascular & renal disease.
- Pts w/ elevated creatinine have increased risk of further postop renal compromise or failure.
  - ➤ Particularly elderly undergoing cardiac or vascular surgery
  - ➤ Use of renal protectants variably successful
  - ➤ Must maintain adequate fluid replacement & intravascular volume
  - ➤ No role for prophylactic dopamine
  - ➤ N-acetyl-cysteine (NAC) for high-risk pts (creatinine >1.5–2.0 mg/dL) undergoing a contrast study such as a cardiac cath, CT; 600 mg bid NAC day of contrast study
- Lower insulin requirements w/ increasing renal insufficiency. If creatinine clearance is 10–50 cc/min, cut insulin in half; if <10 cc/min, lower to 25–50% of normal.
  - ➤ Gastroparesis is common in pts w/ autonomic neuropathy.
    - May have malabsorption process as well
    - Therefore may be at risk for aspiration. Balance fact w/ airway assessment and presence of stiff joint syndrome.

NEUROPSYCHIATRIC

- Increased incidence of depression
- Mood & personality swings may be related to swings in glucose; must rule out & treat hypoglycemia. Identify significant hyperglycemia (>250 mg/dL), ketoacidosis.

EPILEPSY

GEBHARD WAGENER, MD

OVERVIEW

- 10% of the population has a seizure at one point in their life.
- Simple partial seizures: 1 system involved, no loss of consciousness
- Complex partial seizures: >1 system, loss of consciousness possible
- Generalized seizures: always w/ loss of consciousness; either convulsive or nonconvulsive

FLUIDS AND ELECTROLYTES

- Usually unremarkable
- Hyponatremia & hypoglycemia may cause seizures.
- Carbamazepine can cause water retention & hyponatremia.

CARDIOPULMONARY

- Usually unremarkable

HEMATOLOGIC

- Felbamate: aplastic anemia
- Valproic acid: thrombocytopenia, hypofibrinogenemia & dose-related leukopenia

METABOLIC-NUTRITIONAL

- Folate deficiency: phenytoin

GASTROINTESTINAL

- Unremarkable

NEUROPSYCHIATRIC

- Sedation, dyskinesias, ataxia w/ all anti-epileptics

GERIATRIC PATIENT

HUGH R. PLAYFORD, MD

OVERVIEW

N/A

FLUIDS AND ELECTROLYTES

- Progressive decline in renal function w/ age
  - ➤ Vulnerable to fluid overload
  - ➤ Prone to accumulation of drugs/toxins dependent on renal metabolism/excretion
- Decreased renal blood flow, decreased glomerular filtration rate (both parallel decline in cardiac output)
- Serum creatinine often normal or low even in the presence of significant renal dysfunction (less muscle mass & turnover w/ aging)
- Decreased urinary concentrating ability
  - ➤ Decreased ability to retain sodium or fluids if hypovolemic
  - ➤ Prone to hyponatremia
  - ➤ Decreased ability to excrete acid urine

CARDIOPULMONARY

- Decreased responsiveness of autonomic nervous system
- Decreased cardiac output (preserved w/ physical fitness)
- Decreased oxygen requirements
- Resting stroke volume largely unchanged
- Less chronotropic & inotropic responsiveness to stress & catecholamines
- Decreased heart rate in general (increased parasympathetic activity, degenerative changes to sinus node and/or cardiac contractility)
- Congestive heart failure common (hypertension, ischemic heart disease)

- Hypertension common (decreased compliance of blood vessels, renovascular causes)
  - Increased systolic & diastolic BP
- General decline in ventilatory function & gas exchange
- Impaired ventilation
  - Decreased lung elasticity (destruction of pulmonary parenchyma), decreased thoracic compliance (calcification of costochondral cartilages)
  - Dorsal kyphosis, increased anterior-to-posterior diameter, decreased chest expansion
  - Increased residual volume, increased functional residual capacity
  - Decreased vital capacity, decreased FEV1
- Progressive hypoxemia w/ age (airway closure, decreased cardiac output w/ increased ventilation-perfusion matching)

HEMATOLOGIC

N/A

METABOLIC-NUTRITIONAL

- Increased incidence of diabetes mellitus (decreased insulin release, insensitivity of receptor to insulin)
- Hypothyroidism (esp. subclinical) common, up to 13% of elderly (esp. females)
- Frequent association w/ arthritis (rheumatoid & osteoarthritis)

GASTROINTESTINAL

- Decreased hepatic blood flow (parallels the decline in cardiac output)
  - Alters clearance of drugs dependent on hepatic elimination
- Decreased gastric emptying

NEUROPSYCHIATRIC

- Progressive decline in CNS activity
- Progressive loss of neurons, esp. in cerebral cortex

- Decline in conduction velocity of peripheral nerves
- Possible decreased number of fibers in spinal cord tracts
- Implication: decreased dosing requirements of injected & inhaled anesthetic agents
- Altered patterns of sleep (decreased slow-wave stage 4)
  - More time in bed, less time asleep, relatively easily aroused
  - Daytime fatigue
  - Poor tolerance of changes in sleep-wake cycle
  - Prone to sleep apnea (related to obstruction, depressant drugs, CNS deterioration)
- Prone to delirium
  - Pathology (eg, myocardial infarction, infection) or pharmacology
  - Sudden onset, fluctuating course over 24 hrs w/ nocturnal exacerbation, decreased consciousness, globally disordered attention, common hallucinations, impaired orientation, unpredictable psychomotor activity, frequently incoherent speech, often related to physical illness or drug toxicity
  - Needs to be distinguished from dementia (insidious onset, stable course over 24 hrs, no change in level of consciousness, usually normal attention, uncommon hallucinations, impaired orientation, usually normal psychomotor activity, difficulty finding words, uncommonly related to physical illness or drug toxicity)

GI DISEASE

GEBHARD WAGENER, MD

OVERVIEW

Upper GI diseases
- Hiatal hernia
- Achalasia

- Esophagitis
- Esophageal infections: Candida
- Gastrinoma
- Gastric ulcer
- Gastric carcinoma
- Pyloric stenosis: pediatrics
- Duodenal ulcer

Lower GI diseases
- Small bowel obstruction
- Irritable bowel disease
- Carcinoid
- Ulcerative colitis
- Crohn's disease
- Pseudomembranous colitis
- Diverticulitis
- Appendicitis
- Colonic obstruction
- Colon carcinoma

Others
- Malabsorption: small bowel
- Maldigestion: pancreas
- Pancreatitis

Patients receiving long-term steroid treatment for ulcerative colitis (less common for Crohn's disease) may develop osteoporosis.

Osteomalacia & osteoporosis are common after gastrojejunostomy (Billroth II) or total gastrectomy: Vitamin D & calcium malabsorption.

FLUIDS AND ELECTROLYTES
- Inadequate intake
  ➤ Dehydration
- Vomiting, gastric fistula or aspiration

- ➤ Hypochloremic metabolic alkalosis
- ➤ Hypokalemia: GI loss & increased renal secretion as a response to alkalosis
- ➤ Dehydration
- ■ Bowel obstruction (severe disturbances more common w/ small bowel obstruction):
  - ➤ Dehydration (fluid sequestered into bowel wall)
  - ➤ Hypokalemia
  - ➤ Possible lactic acidosis in bowel ischemia or perforation (hyperkalemic)
- ■ Diarrhea
  - ➤ Hypochloremic, non-anion gap acidosis
  - ➤ Hypokalemia
  - ➤ Dehydration
- ■ Bowel preparation for colon surgery
  - ➤ Dehydration & metabolic alkalosis
- ■ Pancreatitis
  - ➤ Lactic acidosis, hypocalcemia, dehydration, sepsis

CARDIOPULMONARY

- ■ Dehydration common in most diseases: tachycardia, hypotension, hyperdynamic state
- ■ Hypokalemia common: causing cardiac hyperpolarization, conduction delays, re-entry & ectopic tachycardia
- ■ Carcinoid
  - ➤ Serotonin, kinins & histamine release: vasoconstriction or vasodilation
  - ➤ Cardiac (mostly right ventricular & tricuspid valve) fibrinous plaques
  - ➤ Bronchoconstriction
- ■ Pancreatitis
  - ➤ ARDS
  - ➤ Right pleural effusion
- ■ Increased intra-abdominal pressure

➤ Decreased functional residual capacity
➤ Increased airway pressure w/ positive-pressure ventilation
➤ Hypoxia

HEMATOLOGIC
■ Anemia
➤ Iron deficiency: w/ chronic bleeding ulcer, colonic polyps or tumors
➤ Vitamin B12 (cobalamin) deficiency anemia: megaloblastic: w/ pernicious anemia, sprue or after resection of terminal ileum or gastrectomy
■ Leukocytosis w/ left shift
➤ Perforation, strangulation, diverticulitis

METABOLIC-NUTRITIONAL
■ Malnutrition common w/ any chronic GI diseases
■ Vitamin deficiency: A, B, E, K,B12
■ Malabsorption (small bowel diseases): weight loss, vitamin deficiency, less steatorrhea
■ Maldigestion (pancreatic diseases): marked steatorrhea
■ Diabetes: diarrhea, steatorrhea, mobility disorder, gastroparesis
■ Pts often receive total parenteral nutrition (TPN): sudden cessation of TPN (eg, intraop) can cause marked hypoglycemia: always give glucose-containing infusion & measure blood glucose frequently when stopping TPN.

GASTROINTESTINAL
■ Motility disorders
➤ Achalasia
➤ Diabetic gastroparesis
➤ Acute pseudo-obstruction (Ogilvie)
■ Obstruction
➤ Small bowel obstruction: adhesion, tumor

- ➤ Large bowel obstruction: volvulus, tumor, ischemic colitis, pseudomembranous colitis (Clostridium difficile)
- ➤ Acute intestinal ischemia
- ■ Infectious/Inflammatory
  - ➤ Perforation
  - ➤ Appendicitis
  - ➤ Diverticulitis
  - ➤ Pancreatitis
  - ➤ Inflammatory bowel disease
- ■ Hemorrhagic
  - ➤ Gastric ulcer
  - ➤ Gastric cancer
  - ➤ Duodenal ulcer
  - ➤ Colon carcinoma
  - ➤ Trauma
- ■ Malabsorption
  - ➤ Inflammatory bowel disease
  - ➤ Sprue

NEUROPSYCHIATRIC
- ■ Stress can cause flare up of inflammatory bowel disease.
- ■ Chronic GI disease can lead to anger, shame, depression.

HEMOGLOBINOPATHIES

DOUGLAS B. COURSIN, MD, AND KARL WILLMANN, MD

OVERVIEW
- ■ Anemia secondary to abnormal hemoglobin (>300 variants)
  - ➤ Sickle cell disease
    - • Inherited hemoglobinopathy
      - • Wide range of symptoms & severity
      - • Homozygotes (SS): sickle cell disease; heterozygotes (SA), sickle cell trait
      - • Sickle cell thalassemia (SC)

- Homozygotes (SS disease)
  - Substitution of valine for glutamic acid on the beta-chain
  - 70–98% of RBCs are hemoglobin S.
    - O_2 dissociation curve shifted to the right
    - Polymerization of the Hgb S precipitates sickling, microvascular obstruction, release of inflammatory mediators, diffuse organ injury & sickle cell crisis.
  - Hemolysis & vaso-occlusive crises induce severe, repetitive, accumulative end-organ injury
    - Vaso-occlusive crisis
      - Severe pain
      - Stroke, acute chest syndrome
      - Ischemia of multiple organs
      - Priapism
      - Infection (osteomyelitis)
    - Chronic end-organ damage
      - Stroke
      - Cardiomegaly/CHF
      - Pulmonary fibrosis
      - Pulmonary hypertension
      - Splenic infarction
      - Cholelithiasis
      - Bone infarction
- 8% of African Americans are SA (heterozygotes, sickle cell trait).
  - Diagnosis: hemoglobin electrophoresis
  - Asymptomatic: treat as if they could sickle intraoperatively
  - Usually do not require specific therapy
- Key issues
  - Avoid precipitating crisis
    - Hypothermia

- Acidosis
- Hypotension
- Hypoxemia
- Supportive care advised even for those w/ SA or trait
  - Adequate hydration
  - Judicious consideration of transfusion therapy as needed to decrease hemoglobin S level to <30%; not routinely advocated since it does not necessarily improve outcome
  - Aim to maintain Hct at least 30.
  - Some receive hydroxyurea.
  - Some younger pts w/ extreme symptoms may benefit from bone marrow transplantation.
- Perioperative
  - Early evaluation & in some cases admission to tune up
    - Hydrate
    - Transfuse as needed if Hct < 30 & if symptoms w/ very high Hgb S level
    - Supplemental O_2
    - Avoid respiratory depression & respiratory acidosis.
  - Avoid circulatory deficiency & stasis.
    - Maintain intravascular volume, normothermia, normal acid-base balance, oxygenation.
  - Tourniquets reported by some to be safe to use when indicated
  - No evidence that one anesthetic agent or technique is better than another
  - Postop maneuvers to maintain oxygenation, avoid acidosis, treat pain
- ➤ Thalassemia
  - Represents a number of inherited abnormalities in hemoglobin synthesis & structure

- Major & minor
  - Affects those of Mediterranean/Middle Eastern/ Indian subcontinent descent most commonly
  - Most common hemoglobinopathy
- Beta-thalassemia major (Cooley's anemia) (severe)
  - Rare
  - Unable to form beta-globin chain of hemoglobin; therefore, adult hemoglobin A is not formed
  - Complex process w/ excessive hemoglobin synthesis, multiple complications including jaundice, hepatosplenomegaly & risk of infection
  - Hemochromatosis
- Beta-thalassemia minor
  - Heterozygote (trait) state of thalassemia compared to homozygote thalassemia major
  - More common than previously appreciated & far more common than thalassemia major
- Alpha-thalassemia
  - Lack production of alpha chain of hemoglobin
    - Homozygote, uniformly lethal in utero or as neonate
    - Heterozygote (trait)
    - Mild anemia, usually microcytic & hypochromic
    - Occasional pts have significant hemolysis & may need splenectomy.
    - Occasionally require transfusion therapy
- Sickle thalassemia disease
  - Usually less severe than SS disease or thalassemia major but more symptomatic than SA (trait)
  - Anemia mild: Hgb 10–12 g/dL
  - Still at risk for veno-occlusive crises
- Anesthetic priorities in thalassemia
  - Depend on severity of disease
  - If pt is transfusion-dependent, evaluate heart & liver function carefully because of potential iron toxicity.

- Extramedullary hematopoiesis may cause enlarged facial bones, resulting in difficult airway mgt & laryngoscopy.
- Anemia secondary to enzyme abnormalities
  - G6PD
    - Affects 10% of African Americans, mainly males
      - Wide variation in enzyme function
    - Chronic hemolysis
    - Drugs that form peroxides by interacting w/ oxyhemoglobin may trigger.
      - May lead to DIC
      - Anesthetic agents do not trigger.
      - Main concerns over antibiotics (sulfa, PCN, INH, nitrofurantoins, antimalarials), also acetaminophen, methylene blue, possibly nitroprusside & others

For a more complete listing, see a standard hematology or pharmacology text.

FLUID AND ELECTROLYTES
N/A

CARDIOPULMONARY
N/A

HEMATOLOGIC
N/A

METABOLIC/NUTRITIONAL
N/A

GASTROINTESTINAL
N/A

NEUROPSYCHIATRIC
N/A

HEMOPHILIA A & HEMOPHILIA B

KARL WILLMANN, MD, AND D. B. COURSIN, MD

OVERVIEW

- Both Hemophilia A & B are X-linked recessive disorders of coagulation. Hemophilia A is a deficit of factor VIII or defective factor VIII. Hemophilia B is either a deficiency or nonfunctional factor IX. In both diseases, severity depends on the level of circulating functional factors.
- Hemophilia A & B
  - Mild: 5–25% normal factor VIII/IX levels
  - Moderate: 1–4% normal factor VIII/IX levels
  - Severe: 0 to <1% normal factor VIII/IX levels
- Severe disease can result in hemarthroses, usually of the larger joints (knee, hip, shoulder, elbow & ankles). There is usually no excessive bleeding w/ minor cuts. Severe disease can also cause muscle hemorrhages & easy bruising. Pts can also have life-threatening intracranial hemorrhage
- Hemophilia A occurs in 1/10,000 male infants.
- Hemophilia B occurs in 1/25,000–50,000 male infants.
- Goals for anesthesia are to increase deficient factors to high enough levels to prevent excessive bleeding both intraop & postop.

FLUID & ELECTROLYTES

- No special concerns

CARDIOPULMONARY

- No special concerns

HEMATOLOGIC

- Deficient or defective clotting factors, causing coagulopathy. Pts have normal platelet & PT but prolonged PTT. One cannot distinguish between hemophilia A & B except by factor analysis. Pts w/ mild disease may not be recognized until surgery or trauma. History of excessive bleeding w/ dental work, heavy menses, epistaxis & lacerations w/ elevated PTT warrant further evaluation for possible hemophilia.

METABOLIC-NUTRITIONAL
N/A

GASTROINTESTINAL
- Pts who have required blood transfusion & factor therapy in the past are at risk for HIV & hepatitis B & C infections & the sequelae of those diseases.
- Pts can have GI bleeds.
- Pts may have hematuria & obstructive symptoms w/ renal dysfunction.
- Follow Bun/Cr/urinalysis.

NEUROPSYCHIATRIC
- Pts may have chronic pain & narcotic dependency after repeated joint hemarthroses.
- Pts are also at risk for spontaneous intracranial hemorrhage.

HERBAL THERAPY

JONATHAN T. KETZLER, MD

OVERVIEW
- Herbal medications are biochemically active compounds that may interact w/ drugs used by anesthesiologists.
- Herbal remedies are not subject to testing by the FDA.
- Lack of herbal standardization makes definitive diagnosis of herb-anesthesia interaction difficult.
- American public spends $5 billion on alternative medicine.

- Compounds are used to fight depression, raise energy levels & improve memory.
- While 22% of pts take herbal meds, only 7 out of 10 tell their doctors.
- ASA advises pts to stop herbal meds 2 wks prior to surgery.
- ASA advises pts who continue to take herbal meds to bring the bottle to surgery.

FLUID & ELECTROLYTES
N/A

CARDIOPULMONARY
N/A

HEMATOLOGIC
N/A

METABOLIC/NUTRITIONAL
N/A

GASTROINTESTINAL
N/A

NEUROPSYCHIATRIC
N/A

HIV & AIDS

GEBHARD WAGENER, MD

OVERVIEW
N/A

FLUIDS AND ELECTROLYTES
- No special care unless diarrhea, vomiting: hypochloremic alkalosis

- Nephropathy w/ proteinuria possible

CARDIOPULMONARY

- Pulmonary: PCP pneumonia, lung abscess, TB, bacterial pneumonias (Pseudomonas, streptococcal pneumonia)
- Cardiac
  - ➤ Myocarditis (toxoplasmosis, Cryptosporidiae, CMV, Coxsackie B virus)
  - ➤ Pericardial effusion common (25%)
  - ➤ Abnormal echocardiogram in 50% of pts w/ AIDS
  - ➤ Endocarditis, left ventricular dysfunction

HEMATOLOGIC

- Neutropenia, immunosuppression
- Anemia
- Thrombocytopenia

METABOLIC-NUTRITIONAL

Often malnutrition: AIDS wasting syndrome

GASTROINTESTINAL

- Diarrhea, nausea, vomiting common
- GI infections: CMV, Herpes, Candida

NEUROPSYCHIATRIC

- AIDS dementia: increased sensitivity to benzodiazepines, opioids
- Neoplasm & infections common: Cryptosporidiae, toxoplasmosis, progressive multifocal leukoencephalopathy: increased ICP possible
- More likely to develop extrapyramidal symptoms from neuroleptics
- Polyneuropathy: distal & symmetric

HYPERTENSION

MUHAMMED ITANI, MD, AND JONATHAN T. KETZLER, MD

OVERVIEW

- Definition: systemic BP > 140/90 on 3 separate measurements
- Essential hypertension accounts for >95% of pts.
- Secondary hypertension accounts for <5%; causes:
  - ➤ Oral contraceptive pills: most common cause in females
  - ➤ Excessive alcohol consumption: most common cause in males
  - ➤ Renovascular hypertension: most common secondary hypertension overall
  - ➤ Pheochromocytoma
  - ➤ Cushing's disease
  - ➤ Conn's syndrome
  - ➤ Aortic coarctation
  - ➤ Hyperthyroidism
- Hypertension is the most important risk factor for cerebral stroke.
- CAD is the most common cause of death in untreated hypertension.
- Hypertension is the major cause of congestive heart failure, arterial aneurysms & end-stage renal disease.
- Hypertensive crisis: acute diastolic BP increase above 130 mm Hg; the urgency for treatment is defined by the rate of BP increase
- Hypertension is common in diabetics & highly associated w/ diabetic nephropathy.

FLUIDS AND ELECTROLYTES

- Hypertensive pts tend to be hypovolemic due to:
  - ➤ Vascular constriction & compensated decreased intravascular volume

> Diuretic-induced intravascular fluid depletion
- Conn's disease: may have hypernatremia & hypokalemia
- May have hyperkalemia w/ ACE inhibitor therapy & hypokalemia w/ diuretic therapy (except w/ spironolactone), but no increased risk for cardiac arrhythmias is seen

CARDIOPULMONARY

- Hypertension can be caused by obstructive sleep apnea; 30% of older or obese pts have sleep-disordered breathing.
- Renovascular disease: upper abdominal bruit may be present; can confirm diagnosis by MRA
- Concentric cardiac hypertrophy & LV wall thickening
- Diastolic dysfunction of varying degrees depends on the severity & chronicity of BP elevation; eventually both systolic & diastolic dysfunction may take place.
- LV hypertrophy predisposes to myocardial ischemia & infarction.

HEMATOLOGIC
N/A

METABOLIC-NUTRITIONAL

- 40% of pts w/ essential hypertension have high serum cholesterol levels (>200 mg/dL).
- Pts may have insulin resistance, dyslipidemia diabetes & obesity.
- 50% of pts have glucose intolerance.
- Progressive loss of renal function occurs w/ poorly controlled hypertension.
- Primary hyperaldosteronism (Conn's syndrome): hypertension, hypernatremia, hypokalemia
- CT scan or MRI shows hyperplastic glands or adrenal gland adenoma.
- Pheochromocytoma is a rare cause of secondary hypertension w/ episodic swings in BP or sustained markedly increased BP.

GASTROINTESTINAL

N/A

NEUROPSYCHIATRIC

- History of cerebrovascular disease (carotid artery stenosis) w/ subsequent stroke or TIAs
- Increased sympathetic nervous system tone
- Encephalopathy may develop in chronic hypertensives if diastolic BP >150 mm Hg; parturient may develop encephalopathy at a diastolic BP <100 mm Hg.
- Shift of the autoregulation curve to the right; this may be reversed w/ volatile anesthetics & ACE inhibitor treatment

---

ICU PATIENT SCHEDULED FOR INTERCURRENT SURGERY

DOUGLAS B. COURSIN, MD

OVERVIEW

- Focus on type of critical illness/unit.
  - ➤ Tailor pt's needs for specific problems.
  - ➤ Organ-specific
    - CCU, Neuro, CT surg, Pediatric
    - Emergent ops for cardiac surgery from CCU & CT surg
      - Organ-specific issues
      - Pacer
      - Assist devices
      - Recent antithrombotics/lytics/anticoagulants
      - Anti-dysrhythmic drugs
  - ➤ General
    - Med-surg
- Critically ill pts commonly require anesthesia care.
  - ➤ • Sedation/analgesic/paralytic meds
    - Pain-sparing procedures & blocks
    - Transport

- Angiographic procedures: radiology, cath lab
- General anesthesia in or out of OR
  - Bedside procedure
  - Provision of inhaled anesthesia for severe reactive airway disease
- Wide age range
- Does the procedure need to be done out of the ICU?
  - Are there alternatives if the pt is deemed too unstable?
  - Could the same or lesser procedure be safely performed in the ICU w/ adequate result?
    - Percutaneous trach
    - Percutaneous feeding tube placement
    - Drainage/irrigation
- Preemptive care is crucial.
  - What was pt's premorbid state of health?
    - Nursing home pts may be more prone to colonization w/ resistant organisms.
    - Comorbid pathology may direct preventive modalities & selection of monitoring & guide prognosis.
    - Key areas
      - CV risk stratification
      - Underlying pulmonary reserve
      - Renal compromise
      - Hepatic reserve
        - Synthetic function
        - Albumin
      - Immune status
        - Is pt immunocompetent?
        - Acquired vs. inherited immunocompromise
      - Endocrinopathy: intrinsic or acquired
        - Diabetes mellitus
        - Adrenal insufficiency
        - Panhypopituitarism
        - Thyroid dysfunction

- Why is the pt in the ICU?
- How long has the pt been there?
- Review pt's problem list, since crucial pieces of info may be overlooked w/out a systematic review.
- What is the mechanism of injury?
  - Trauma vs. other
- Organ system review
  - CNS
    - Mental status
    - Baseline neuro function, esp. in elderly, CNS infected & those w/ neurovascular compromise, stroke, hypoperfusion, trauma
      - What meds is the pt receiving that may alter mental status?
      - Is the pt on anticonvulsants? Might the pt need anticonvulsants perioperatively?
        - How might these affect anesthesia meds, effect on paralytics?
      - What is the pt's need for ICP meds?
        - Osmotics
        - Loop diuretics
        - Barbiturate therapy
  - CV
    - Previous MI
      - Cardiac reserve
      - Recent echo, invasive monitoring
      - CHF
      - Diastolic dysfunction
      - Has the pt recently received antithrombotic or anticoagulant meds?
    - Baseline rhythm
      - Sinus vs. other
      - Intermittent rhythm
      - Risk for atrial fib

- Risk for heart block or conduction delay
- Need for external or internal pacemaker
- Presence of pacemaker/AICD
  - External
  - Internal
  - Type & mode
  - Plan for what to do in OR
- Assessment of cardiac function
  - Invasive/noninvasive modalities
  - UO, hemodynamics, SvO_2, gastric tonometry, lactate, acid-base, etc.
- Therapies altering cardiac function
  - Mechanical (IABP, VAD, ECMO)
  - Pharmacological (sympathetic agonists & antagonists, vasopressors, ACE inhibitors, PDE inhibitors, etc.)
- Pulmonary
  - Smoker
  - Chronic disease
  - Infectious
  - Airway assessment (presence of an artificial airway, difficulty of establishing airway [eg, facial trauma])
  - Ventilated: invasive vs. noninvasive vs. partial, such as nighttime CPAP or BiPAP
  - Gas exchange PaO_2/FiO_2
  - Will pt need a unique form of ventilatory support, pressure control, oscillation, high frequency, other?
    - Is this available in OR?
  - Pharmacological therapies
    - Sympathomimetics, anticholinergics, antimuscarinics, steroids (systemic or inhaled), antimicrobials

- Pulmonary side effects (opioids, beta antagonists)
- Hepatic
  - Synthetic function
  - Immune function
  - Hepatitis
    - Active
    - Old
  - Liver function tests
    - Hepatocellular enzymes: ALT, AST
    - Hepatic synthesis: INR, albumin
    - Canalicular: alk phos, bilirubin, GGT
- Renal
  - Adequate reserve
  - External support (eg, IHD, CVVHDF, peritoneal dialysis), frequency, adequacy
  - Diuretics
  - Nephrotoxic agents
  - Function
    - Urinalysis
    - Culture
    - Creatinine, estimated clearance

■ Therapies requiring continuation outside the ICU need to be assessed.
  ➤ Ventilation
  ➤ Cardiovascular support
  ➤ Renal replacement therapies can often be suspended intraoperatively.
  ➤ Anticoagulation (systemic, regional [eg, w/ dialysis])
  ➤ Antimicrobials
  ➤ Withhold activated protein C if there is a prospect of interventional therapy.
  ➤ Analgesics & sedatives

➤ Nutritional support may require modification (eg, replacement of enteral nutrition w/ IV dextrose).

■ Must provide level of care at least equal to ICU during transport & while out of ICU in OR or radiology or during outside intervention

■ Does pt require isolation?
  ➤ Why?
  ➤ Resistant infection
  ➤ Biologic/chemical exposure
  ➤ Other

■ Despite our best efforts, ICU pts have significantly higher morbidity & mortality than non-ICU pts.
  ➤ Discuss w/ surgeon/radiologist/cardiologist prior to procedure.
  ➤ Discuss w/ family.

■ Clarify code status.
  ➤ DNR
  ➤ Suspended during procedure

■ Ensure adequacy of:
  ➤ Consent
  ➤ Handover from ICU staff
  ➤ Blood product availability
  ➤ Monitoring
  ➤ Therapies at destination (ventilator, number of pumps, infusions, etc.)

FLUID AND ELECTROLYTES

■ Current maintenance
■ Current need for ongoing resuscitation
  ➤ Hypovolemia
  ➤ Bleed
  ➤ Distributive shock such as sepsis
  ➤ Spinal shock

- ➤ Recent burn
- ➤ Ongoing third-space losses related to open wounds, fistulae, etc.
- ■ Identify electrolyte abnormalities & current therapy.
  - ➤ Hyponatremia
    - Dilutional
    - Total body
    - SIADH
    - Cerebral salt-wasting process
    - Current level & anticipated rate of correction
    - Take into account what intraoperative fluids will do to correct this & possibility of overly rapid correction.
  - ➤ Hypernatremia
    - Diabetes insipidus
    - Hypovolemia: total body salt status
      - Need for salt & water
    - Calculate free water deficit.
    - Take into account what intraoperative fluids will do to correct this & possibility of overly rapid correction.
  - ➤ Hyperkalemia
    - Spurious vs. real: hemolysis
    - Renal function
    - Potassium-containing solutions
    - Potassium-sparing meds
      - Diuretics: spironolactone
      - ACE inhibitors
    - ECG changes
  - ➤ Hypokalemia
    - ECG changes
    - Clinical context
      - Diuretics
      - Diuresis
    - What is the degree?
      - Calculate total body deficit.

- How fast do you need to correct?
  - Monitoring
    - ECG
    - Frequent serum potassium levels
- Hypermagnesemia
  - Renal function
  - Exogenous administration
- Hypomagnesemia
  - Diuretics
  - Aminoglycosides
  - Diarrhea
  - Diabetes
  - Other meds
  - Rhythm
- Hyperphosphatemia
  - Renal function
  - Calcium
  - Calcium × phosphorus >75, possible metastatic deposits of calcium phosphate
- Hypophosphatemia
  - Degree
  - Risk for rhabdomyolysis
  - Weakness
  - Etiology
    - COPD
    - Nutritional
- Hyperchloremia
  - Has pt received large saline volumes & does pt have a non-anion gap acidosis?
- Hypochloremia
  - Diuretic-induced
  - High NG losses
- Hypercalcemia
  - Malignancy

- PTH
- Resorption
- What is the phosphorus level?
- What is the calcium-phosphorus index?
- Excessive ingestion/infusion
➤ Hypocalcemia
- Renal function
- Postop
- Diuretics
- What is the QTc on the ECG?
  - What drugs is pt receiving that might prolong the QTc & increase the chance of torsades de pointes?
■ Evaluate current acid-base balance.
➤ Is there a metabolic, respiratory or combined acidosis or alkalosis?
- Does it need to be corrected preop?
- Is the procedure likely to exacerbate this?
  - Need for high minute ventilation
  - Lactic acid production/undermetabolism
- Does pt require $NaCO_3$, THAM, ongoing dialysis, other?

CARDIOPULMONARY
■ Hemodynamic assessment
➤ Blood pressure
➤ Rhythm
➤ Rate
■ Risk
➤ Ischemia: demand or myocardium at risk
➤ Acute coronary syndrome
➤ Recent MI
■ Type of hemodynamic monitoring & access, ongoing or anticipated
➤ Is it sufficient for the anticipated procedure?
➤ Do you need to intensify level of hemodynamic monitoring or access?

- ➤ Arterial catheter
- ➤ CVP/PAC
- ➤ PICC
- ➤ Echocardiographic
- ➤ Noninvasive cardiac output
- ■ Need for vasopressors
  - ➤ Dose & mode of delivery
    - Pump type & compatibility w/ anesthesia systems
    - Adequacy of infusion; do you need another bag of the infusion?
  - ➤ Inotrope
  - ➤ Vasoconstrictor
  - ➤ Vasodilator
- ■ Need for rate or rhythm control
  - ➤ Dose, mode of delivery, adequacy of drug
    - Beta blocker
    - Calcium channel blocker
    - Amiodarone
    - Antidysrhythmic
      - Lidocaine
      - Procainamide
      - Other
    - Is the pt paced?
      - Temporary
        - Internal
        - External
      - Permanent
        - Mode
        - Programmable
        - Do you need to integrate the pacer & place into a default mode prior to surgery or exposure to cautery?
- ■ Is there an AICD in place? What is its status & does it need to be modified for the perioperative period?
- ■ Is an assist device in place?

➤ Are you organized to transport w/ the device & have it function out of the ICU?

■ Is an assist device possibly required?
➤ IABP
➤ LVAD/RVAD

■ What is the pt's respiratory status?
➤ How tenuous is the pt?
➤ What is the pt's baseline pulmonary function/reserve?
➤ Recent ABG
➤ With the current respiratory status, will be it adequate for the procedure planned? Can the status be improved or modified to tolerate the procedure?

■ What is the mode of ventilation?
➤ Invasive
➤ Noninvasive
➤ Can you reproduce the mode of ventilation in the OR, or do you need an ICU ventilator placed in the OR?
➤ What are the ventilator settings?
➤ Can you adequately ventilate the pt on transfer?
  • Attempt Ambu bag w/ PEEP prior to transfer.
  • If above is unsuccessful, use transfer ventilator or abort.

HEMATOLOGIC

■ Is the pt anemic? Leukopenic? Thrombocytopenic? Pancytopenic?
➤ Does the pt require protective isolation?

■ Does the pt have blood type & cross-matched or screened?
➤ Does the pt need specialized blood products?
  • Irradiated
  • Filtered
  • HLA-typed
➤ Does the pt have an antibody?
  • Anti-I & cold antibodies require warmed blood.

■ Has the pt been transfused before?

- Has the pt consented to transfusion?
- Is the pt's oxygen delivery adequate?
- Does the pt require transfusion preop or intraop?
  - Red cells
  - Platelets
  - Plasma
  - Specialized blood components
- Does the pt have DIC or an inherited coagulopathy?
  - Coags: INR, aPTT
  - Platelets
  - Need for replacement factors
- Is the pt receiving drugs associated w/ bleeding or clotting? If stopped, when?
  - Antiplatelets
  - Antithrombotics
  - Anticoagulants, including activated protein C
  - Lytic agents
  - Plasminogen inhibitors
- Does the pt have heparin-induced thrombocytopenia (antibody)?
- Does the pt have hemolysis?
  - Smear
  - Bilirubin, hemosiderin, haptoglobin

METABOLIC-NUTRITIONAL

- Is the pt hypermetabolic?
  - Fever
  - Sepsis/infection
- Is the pt overfed?
  - High carbohydrate load
- Could the pt have a refeeding syndrome?
  - Recent starvation/malnourishment
  - Hypokalemia
- What is the status of the nutritional supplementation?
  - IV dextrose

➤ IV TPN
➤ Enteric nutrition
➤ Does the nutritional delivery need to be modified for the procedure?
  • Eg, change the enteric nutrition to IV
  • Care to maintain blood sugars, especially if using insulin

GASTROINTESTINAL

■ Is the pt at risk for stress ulceration?
  ➤ Has the pt had a GI bleed?
  ➤ Does the pt have varices?
■ Is the pt receiving acid suppression?
  ➤ H2 blocker
  ➤ Proton pump inhibitor
■ Does the pt have altered GI motility?
  ➤ NG in place
  ➤ Ileus
  ➤ Aspiration risk
  ➤ Recent tube feedings
■ Does the pt have diarrhea?
  ➤ Etiology
■ Hepatic function
  ➤ Adequacy of hepatic synthetic function
    • Glucose
    • Protein
    • Coag factors
  ➤ Does the pt have active hepatitis?
  ➤ Drug metabolism
    • Volume of distribution
    • Drug clearance
■ Renal
■ What is the pt's baseline renal function?
  ➤ How much urine does the pt make?

➤ Does the pt respond to diuretics?

➤ Is the pt adequately hydrated?

➤ What is the pt's risk for postop renal insufficiency/failure?

- Diabetes mellitus
- Age
- CHF, low cardiac output, hypotension, hypovolemia
- Ongoing nephrotoxic agents
- Baseline renal compromise

➤ Is acute, acute-on-chronic, or chronic dysfunction or failure present?

■ Does the pt require dialytic support?

➤ Hemodialysis

➤ Renal replacement therapy

➤ Peritoneal

■ How recently was the pt dialyzed? What are the most recent lytes & acid-base status?

■ Will the pt need dialytic support during surgery?

■ Do drug doses need to be altered because of low GFR?

NEUROPSYCHIATRIC

■ Delirium is common.

■ Is the pt on sedatives/antipsychotic meds?

■ Depression: antidepressants, MAOIs, amphetamines

■ Drug interactions

IDIOPATHIC HYPERTROPHIC SUBAORTIC STENOSIS (IHSS)

ROBERT N. SLADEN, MD

OVERVIEW

■ Etiology

➤ Autosomal dominant inheritance

> Variable penetrance
- Variable onset, slow progression, manifests in second to fourth decade
- Key symptoms similar to aortic stenosis
  > Angina
  > Syncope or presyncope
  > Sudden death (during exertion)

FLUID & ELECTROLYTES
N/A

CARDIOPULMONARY
- Hemodynamic profile: hypodynamic
- Left ventricle (LV) undergoes asymmetric hypertrophy (pressure overload)
  > EF is increased >0.7 (end-systolic collapse).
  > Restricted forward cardiac output: impaired circulatory reserve, effort intolerance, dyspnea
  > Syncope or sudden death may occur w/ LV outflow tract (LVOT) obstruction.
- Mitral regurgitation
  > Rapid systolic ejection creates Venturi effect in aortic outflow tract.
  > Pulls mitral valve anterior during systole (systolic anterior motion [SAM])
  > Degree of SAM & mitral regurgitation very variable
- Impaired myocardial oxygen balance (MVO_2)
  > Increased demand (increased afterload, contractility)
  > Decreased supply (decreased aortic diastolic pressure, thickened myocardium)
  > Angina may occur w/out coronary artery disease (CAD).
  > Earlier-onset angina w/ concomitant CAD
- Diagnosis

- ➤ Rapid, short-lived upstroke to pulse (reflects aortic ejection)
- ➤ Pansystolic murmur radiating to axilla (mitral regurgitation)
- ➤ Cardiomegaly on chest radiograph
- ➤ Left ventricular hypertrophy (LVH) on ECG
- ➤ Increasing gradient across aortic valve (critical: peak >70 mm Hg, mean >50 mm Hg)
- ➤ Decreasing aortic valve area (normal 2–4 cm^2, critical <1.0 cm^2)
- ■ Acute decompensation (low cardiac output syndrome)
  - ➤ Acute atrial fibrillation, tachyarrhythmias (loss of atrial kick)
- ■ Late manifestations
  - ➤ Congestive heart failure
  - ➤ Sudden death
- ■ Increased risk of perioperative myocardial ischemia
  - ➤ Acute ischemia w/ relatively mild perturbations
  - ➤ Low cardiac output syndrome (unable to respond to postop demands)
  - ➤ Cardiac arrest: CPR may be unsuccessful in overcoming LVOT obstruction

HEMATOLOGIC
N/A

METABOLIC/NUTRITIONAL
N/A

GASTROINTESTINAL
N/A

NEUROPSYCHIATRIC
N/A

ISCHEMIC HEART DISEASE

MUHAMMED ITANI, MD, AND JONATHAN T. KETZLER, MD

OVERVIEW

- Leading cause of death & health care expenditure in USA
- Major cause of morbidity & loss of productivity
- May be present in up to 30% of older pts undergoing surgery
- Cardiac dysrhythmias are the major cause of sudden death.
- Risk factors: male gender, increasing age, hypercholesterolemia, hypertension, cigarette smoking, diabetes mellitus, obesity, sedentary lifestyle, family history of premature ischemic heart disease (male <55 yrs of age, female <65 yrs)
- Initial manifestations: angina pectoris, MI or sudden death

FLUID & ELECTROLYTES

N/A

CARDIOPULMONARY

- Pathophysiology: narrowing of coronary arteries by plaques; plaque rupture; acute thrombus; & myocardial oxygen supply/demand mismatch
- Manifestations: angina pectoris, acute MI or sudden death
- Sudden death due to dysrhythmias
- Angina pectoris
  - ➤ Can be caused by coronary artery atherosclerosis, endothelial damage or coronary vasospasm (variant or Prinzmetal's angina)
  - ➤ Can be stable (reproducible w/ same extent of effort) or unstable (new onset, occurs w/ less effort, occurs at rest)
  - ➤ Symptoms: retrosternal chest discomfort w/ radiation to neck, lower jaw, left shoulder & arm, back, right upper extremity & epigastrium
  - ➤ Symptoms can be exacerbated by stress & relieved by rest or nitroglycerine.

➤ Position or direct pressure does not affect symptoms.
➤ Symptoms last up to 30 min.
➤ Pts w/ stable angina may benefit from pharmacologic treatment only (see below).
➤ Pts w/ unstable angina or severe anginal symptoms may require nonpharmacologic treatment (revascularization w/ angioplasty or surgery).
➤ Acute myocardial infarction (AMI)
- Caused by coronary artery plaque rupture & consequent lumen occlusion by platelet aggregation & thrombin deposition
- Mortality significantly decreased by early reperfusion therapy (thrombolytic therapy, angioplasty & stenting within 12 hrs of onset)
- Prognosis is determined by residual LV function, dysrhythmias & residual ischemia.
- Mortality is highest within the first 3 months after onset.
- LV function can improve within the first 3 months & must be measured after 3 months to determine long-term prognosis.
- Pts may present w/ signs & symptoms of chest pain, apprehension, hypotension, tachycardia, LV or RV failure, signs of congestive heart failure, dysrhythmias, new-onset murmur due to ischemic mitral valve regurgitation.
- Complications may include ventricular dysrhythmias, atrial fibrillation, heart block, pericarditis, ischemic mitral regurgitation, ventricular septal defect, cardiac rupture & tamponade, congestive heart failure, right ventricular infarction, CVA.

HEMATOLOGIC
■ Relative lymphocytopenia w/ AMI
■ Reactive leukocytosis w/ AMI

METABOLIC-NUTRITIONAL

■ Diabetes mellitus is the most common endocrine disorder associated w/ IHD.

■ Pts w/ diabetes may have blunted or no symptoms associated w/ IHD (silent ischemia, silent MI).

■ Pts on beta blockers may have masked sympathetic response to hypoglycemia.

■ Improved glucose control improves the outcome after AMI.

GASTROINTESTINAL

■ Epigastric discomfort

■ AMI may be associated w/ nausea & vomiting.

■ Diffuse esophageal spasm may mimic symptoms of angina pectoris & may be relieved w/ nitroglycerine.

■ Concomitant peripheral vascular disease may affect the mesenteric arteries & cause abdominal angina.

■ GI bleeding as a complication of anticoagulant and/or thrombolytic therapy

NEUROPSYCHIATRIC

■ CVA due to:
  ➤ Concomitant cerebrovascular disease
  ➤ Embolization of LV thrombus that forms w/ anterior & apical MI

■ Intracerebral hemorrhage as a complication of thrombolytic therapy, esp. in elderly & hypertensive pts during the first 24 hrs after treatment

■ Mental stress may accompany silent angina.

■ Depression

LATEX ALLERGY

ARTHUR ATCHABAHIAN, MD

OVERVIEW

■ Risk factors

- ➤ Healthcare worker
- ➤ Spina bifida
- ➤ Multiple surgeries
- ➤ Cerebral palsy
- ➤ History of allergy to fruits such as banana, avocado, papaya, kiwi, chestnuts
- ■ Any reaction to latex (eg, balloons, dental care), including:
  - ➤ Contact dermatitis
  - ➤ Rhinitis
  - ➤ Conjunctivitis
  - ➤ Respiratory reaction
  - ➤ Anaphylaxis should be considered as a sign of latex allergy.
- ■ Any history of unexplained intraoperative anaphylaxis, especially if not concomitant w/ induction, is strongly suggestive; pt should be treated as if having documented latex allergy.

FLUIDS AND ELECTROLYTES
Normal unless anaphylaxis occurs

CARDIOPULMONARY
- ■ Normal w/out crisis
- ■ Anaphylaxis in a crisis, w/:
  - ➤ Vasodilation
  - ➤ Capillary leak
  - ➤ Bronchospasm
  - ➤ Up to cardiovascular collapse & cardiac arrest

HEMATOLOGIC
Normal, possible eosinophilia

METABOLIC-NUTRITIONAL
Normal except for possible fruit allergy (see overview)

GASTROINTESTINAL
Normal

NEUROPSYCHIATRIC
Pts w/ spina bifida or cerebral palsy are at increased risk.

LIVER DISEASE

ROBERT N. SLADEN, MD

OVERVIEW

N/A

FLUID & ELECTROLYTES

- Primary concerns: refractory edema & ascites
- Hypoalbuminemia + portal hypertension = ascites + intravascular hypovolemia
- Secondary hyperaldosteronism
  - Salt & water retention
  - Potassium loss
  - Hypokalemic metabolic alkalosis
  - Generalized edema (anasarca)
  - Progressive ascites, resistant to loop diuretics
- Consequences of ascites
  - Decreased FRC
  - Atelectasis
  - Hypoxemia
  - Decreased venous return & renal blood flow (RBF)
  - Spontaneous bacterial peritonitis (10% of pts)

CARDIOPULMONARY

- Primary concerns: hyperdynamic circulation, hypoxemia
- Hyperdynamic circulation w/ fixed low systemic vascular resistance (SVR)
- AV shunts in skin (nevi, erythema), GI tract, lung
- Impaired circulatory reserve (hypovolemia, sepsis, myocardial ischemia)
- Alcoholic cardiomyopathy (cirrhosis w/ or w/out thiamine deficiency)
- Hepatopulmonary syndrome
  - Hypoxemia (AV shunts), atelectasis

➤ Rarely pulmonary hypertension
➤ Orthodeoxia: SpO_2 decreases when upright
■ Postop acute respiratory failure
➤ Pulmonary edema (hypoalbuminemia)
➤ Atelectasis (ascites)
➤ Pneumonia (aspiration, impaired resistance)

HEMATOLOGIC

■ Primary concerns: factor VII deficiency, thrombocytopenia
➤ Factor VII deficiency
➤ Prolonged PT (impaired synthesis, vitamin K absorption)
■ Thrombocytopenia
➤ Hypersplenism (portal hypertension), bleeding, DIC
■ Factor V deficiency
➤ Acute marker after orthotopic liver transplantation
■ Dysfibrinogenemia (abnormal fibrinogen synthesis)
➤ Fibrinogen level may be normal.
■ Macrocytic anemia
➤ Alcohol-induced bone marrow suppression

METABOLIC-NUTRITIONAL

■ Primary concerns: hypoglycemia, malnutrition, infection
➤ Hypoglycemia (acute hepatic failure, end-stage liver disease)
➤ Failure to synthesize glycogen
■ Kwashiorkor (hypoalbuminemic protein malnutrition)
➤ Catabolic effects of hepatic failure
➤ Depleted lean body mass
➤ Hypoalbuminemia
➤ Low colloid oncotic pressure (COP)
➤ Exacerbates edema, ascites
■ Immunocompromise
➤ Liver failure, malnutrition
➤ Nosocomial, opportunistic infections
➤ Wound dehiscence, fistulas, bedsores

GASTROINTESTINAL

- Primary concerns: portal hypertension, varices, jaundice
- Potential for active viral hepatitis (A, C, D)
- GI irritation
  - Anorexia, hiccups, nausea, vomiting
  - Delayed gastric emptying (increased risk of regurgitation, aspiration)
  - Exacerbated by severe ascites (increased abdominal pressure)
- Major risk of GI hemorrhage
  - Esophageal, gastric varices (portal hypertension)
  - Hemorrhoids
- Increased risk of peptic ulcer disease (PUD)
  - Differential diagnosis: varices
- Jaundice
  - Late sign, index of obstruction rather than liver failure
  - Exacerbated by renal failure (conjugated hyperbilirubinemia)

Renal

- Primary renal concerns: multifactorial acute renal failure
  - Hepatorenal syndrome
    - Obstructive jaundice (total bilirubin >8 mg/dL) or severe liver failure
    - Portal endotoxemia
    - Intense renal vasoconstriction (vasomotor nephropathy)
    - Prerenal syndrome: oliguria w/ low urine sodium (10 mEq/L or less)
  - Compartment syndrome
    - Tense ascites, increased renal venous pressure
  - Acute tubular necrosis
    - Acute hypovolemia (eg, GI bleeding)
  - Delayed uremia
    - BUN low (even w/ GI bleeding or ARF)

- Failure of hepatic arginine cycle that converts urea to NH_3

NEUROPSYCHIATRIC
- Primary concerns: encephalopathy, neuropathy
- Hepatic encephalopathy
  - Grade 1: confabulation, constructional apraxia
  - Grade 2: drowsiness, asterixis, confusion
  - Grade 3: stupor
  - Grade 4: coma
- Fulminant hepatic failure
  - Coma w/ acute cerebral edema (poor prognosis)
- Precipitating factors for acute encephalopathy
  - Hypovolemia (excessive diuresis)
  - Alkalosis (increased conversion of $NH_4 +$ to $NH_3 +$)
  - GI bleeding, surgery, infection
- Alcohol-induced encephalopathy
  - Thiamine deficiency
  - Wernicke's encephalopathy (oculomotor palsy, cerebellar ataxia)
  - Korsakoff's psychosis (amnesia, confabulation)

MALIGNANT HYPERTHERMIA

HUGH R. PLAYFORD, MD

OVERVIEW
N/A

FLUIDS AND ELECTROLYTES

Without crisis
- Usually unremarkable
- Creatinine kinase may be mildly elevated (poor sensitivity & specificity)

In a crisis

■ Increased cellular metabolism

➤ Increased temperature, carbon dioxide, lactate, acidemia, creatinine kinase, potassium, calcium, myoglobin; later increased BUN

➤ Decreased bicarbonate, oxygen

CARDIOPULMONARY

Without crisis

■ Usually unremarkable

In a crisis

■ Acute pulmonary edema

■ Elevation of end-tidal carbon dioxide

■ Arrhythmias (usually related to hyperkalemia)

HEMATOLOGIC

Without crisis

■ Usually normal

In a crisis

■ DIC

METABOLIC-NUTRITIONAL

Associated conditions

■ Central core disease, Duchenne muscular dystrophy, King-Denborough syndrome, other myopathies (Schwartz-Jampel syndrome, Fukuyama type of muscular dystrophy, Becker muscular dystrophy, periodic paralysis, myotonia congenita, sarcoplasmic reticulum adenosine triphosphatase deficiency, mitochondrial myopathy)

■ Masseter muscle spasm (controversial)

Coincidental conditions

■ Sudden infant death syndrome, neuroleptic malignant syndrome, other diseases (lymphomas, osteogenesis imperfecta, glycogen storage disease)

Without crisis
- Usually normal

In a crisis
- Hypermetabolism, hyperthermia, increased carbon dioxide production, muscular rigidity

GASTROINTESTINAL
N/A

NEUROPSYCHIATRIC
Without crisis
- Usually normal
- May have evidence of associated conditions

In a crisis
- Seizures, coma, muscular rigidity, paralysis

MITRAL REGURGITATION

ROBERT N. SLADEN, MD

OVERVIEW
- Etiology:
  - Rheumatic fever (but less common than mitral stenosis)
  - Mitral valve prolapse
  - Acute or chronic ischemia (papillary muscle dysfunction)
  - Severe dilated cardiomyopathy
- Variable onset, slow progression, manifests in third to sixth decade

FLUID & ELECTROLYTES
N/A

CARDIOPULMONARY
- Hemodynamic profile: hyperdynamic
- Left ventricle undergoes eccentric hypertrophy (volume overload)

> Restricted forward cardiac output: impaired circulatory reserve, effort intolerance, dyspnea
> Afterload is decreased by regurgitation into left atrium.
> This masks impaired function, preserves ejection fraction (EF).
> EF < 0.5 implies ventricular decompensation.

■ Left atrium is exposed to volume, pressure overload
> Pulmonary congestion, edema, hemoptysis
> Atrial fibrillation inevitable w/ time

■ Diagnosis
> Pansystolic murmur radiating to axilla, S3
> V wave on pulmonary artery wedge tracing (may become resorbed w/ time)
> Mitral regurgitation visualized on echo

■ Acute decompensation (acute pulmonary congestion/ edema)
> Acute atrial fibrillation, tachyarrhythmias (loss of atrial kick)

■ Late manifestations
> Cardiac cachexia
> Severe pulmonary hypertension, right ventricular dysfunction, hepatic congestion

■ Increased risk of postop cardiogenic shock, pulmonary edema, atelectasis & pneumonia
> Left ventricle decompensates because afterload increased (left atrial "decanting" removed).
> Residual pulmonary edema
> High risk of postop atrial fibrillation & other arrhythmias

HEMATOLOGIC
■ Chronic atrial fibrillation inevitable w/ time
> Constant risk of intracardiac thrombus & stroke
> Mandates anticoagulation, usually w/ coumadin (INR >2.0)

➤ Will require careful planning for perioperative discontinuation

METABOLIC-NUTRITIONAL
- Cardiac cachexia
  - ➤ Decreased muscle mass
  - ➤ Decreased FRC & ventilatory reserve

GASTROINTESTINAL
N/A

NEUROPSYCHIATRIC
N/A

MITRAL STENOSIS

ROBERT N. SLADEN, MD

OVERVIEW
- Etiology: rheumatic fever (still prevalent in underdeveloped countries)
  - ➤ Slow progression, manifests in third to sixth decade

FLUID & ELECTROLYTES
N/A

CARDIOPULMONARY
- Hemodynamic profile: hypodynamic
- Left ventricle spared, small; brunt borne by left atrium
  - ➤ Restricted cardiac output: impaired circulatory reserve, effort intolerance, dyspnea
  - ➤ Increased left atrial pressure: pulmonary congestion, edema, hemoptysis
  - ➤ Atrial fibrillation inevitable w/ time
- Diagnosis confirmed by finding gradient >10 mm Hg across mitral valve.
  - ➤ Gradient may be relatively low at rest.

- ➤ True severity of mitral stenosis unmasked by tachycardia (increased gradient)
- Acute decompensation (acute pulmonary congestion/edema)
  - ➤ Tachycardia, increased cardiac output (increased pulmonary artery pressure)
  - ➤ Acute atrial fibrillation, tachyarrhythmias
  - ➤ Sepsis, labor & delivery
- Late manifestations
  - ➤ Cardiac cachexia
  - ➤ Severe pulmonary hypertension, right ventricular dysfunction, hepatic congestion
- Increased risk of postop pulmonary edema, atelectasis & pneumonia
  - ➤ Residual pulmonary edema
  - ➤ Risk of "flash" pulmonary edema w/ increased cardiac output

HEMATOLOGIC

- Chronic atrial fibrillation inevitable w/ time
  - ➤ Constant risk of intracardiac thrombus & stroke
  - ➤ Mandates anticoagulation, usually w/ coumadin (INR >2.0)
  - ➤ Will require careful planning for perioperative discontinuation

METABOLIC-NUTRITIONAL

- Cardiac cachexia
  - ➤ Decreased muscle mass
  - ➤ Decreased FRC & ventilatory reserve

GASTROINTESTINAL
N/A

NEUROPSYCHIATRIC
N/A

MORBID OBESITY

HUGH R. PLAYFORD, MD

OVERVIEW
N/A

FLUIDS AND ELECTROLYTES
- Increased blood & plasma volume

CARDIOPULMONARY
- Hypertension
- Increased cardiac output (via stroke volume, not heart rate)
- Pulmonary hypertension (chronic hypoxemia and/or increased blood volume)
- Coronary artery disease (2x risk of non-obese)
- Ventricular hypertrophy and/or dysfunction (left & right)
- Restrictive pulmonary disease (thoracic & abdominal weight loading)
  - Increased work of breathing
- Difficult airway
- Obesity hypoventilation syndrome or Pickwickian syndrome
- Chronic hypoxemia

HEMATOLOGIC
- Hypercoagulability
- Polycythemia (secondary to hypoxemia)

METABOLIC-NUTRITIONAL
- Increased metabolism (increased O_2 consumption, CO_2 production)
- Diabetes mellitus

GASTROINTESTINAL
- Hiatal hernia
- Gastroparesis

- Fatty liver infiltration
- Cholelithiasis

NEUROPSYCHIATRIC
- Psychological disorders

MULTIPLE SCLEROSIS

KARL WILLMANN, MD

OVERVIEW
- Multiple sclerosis (MS) is an autoimmune demyelinating disease that affects both the spinal cord & brain. It does not affect peripheral nerves.
  - Occurs in females more frequently than males
  - More common in Northern Hemisphere
  - More common in Caucasians
- Disease characterized by remission & relapse of symptoms
  - Symptoms may include:
    - Paresthesias
    - Spasticity
    - Optic neuritis
    - Muscular weakness
    - Urinary incontinence
    - Ataxia
  - May be benign w/ mild symptoms & long periods of remission
  - May progress relentlessly w/ permanent symptoms & severe disability, including quadriparesis.
- Pathophysiology is a cycle of CNS inflammation, demyelination & axonal damage w/ plaque formation.
- Diagnosis
  - Clinical findings combined w/ brain imaging
  - MRI: plaques in spine or brain are characteristic of MS

- CSF: increased levels of IgG
- CNS nerve studies: slowed conduction (increased latency on evoked potentials)
- Wide range of symptoms, depending on plaque location
  - Isolated visual disturbances (optic nerve involvement)
  - Spasticity & muscular weakness
  - Gait disturbances
  - Bladder dysfunction
  - Seizure disorders

FLUID AND ELECTROLYTES
- No special concerns from MS itself

CARDIOPULMONARY
- No special concerns from MS itself

HEMATOLOGIC
- No special concerns from MS itself

METABOLIC-NUTRITIONAL
- No special concerns unless disease is severe enough to limit adequate nutritional intake

GASTROINTESTINAL
- Pharyngeal or laryngeal dysfunction (increased risk of aspiration)

NEUROPSYCHIATRIC
- Symptoms depend on the degree of cortex involvement; may include:
  - Emotional disturbance
  - Seizure
  - Memory disturbance
  - Cognitive decline

MUSCULAR DYSTROPHY

JONATHAN T. KETZLER, MD

OVERVIEW

- Muscular dystrophies are a group of primary muscular disorders of unknown cause.
- Often benign in childhood but progress rapidly w/ age
- Duchenne's muscular dystrophy is the most common & severe type.
- Characterized by degeneration of muscle fibers w/ infiltration by fat & fibrous tissue
- Early symptoms of weakness in proximal muscles & muscles of the pelvic girdle
- Typically begins btwn ages 2 & 7
- Becker's dystrophy is similar to Duchenne's but onset is later & progression slower.
- Fascioscapulohumeral dystrophy & limb-girdle dystrophy come on in adulthood & are not nearly as severe.

FLUID & ELECTROLYTES
N/A

CARDIOPULMONARY

- Cardiac muscle is involved w/ dystrophic process.
- Almost all pts have some cardiac abnormality, but only 10% are clinically significant.
- Diastolic dysfunction is present in >80% of pts.
- Ejection fraction is decreased in 21% of pts.
- Most pts do not have cardiovascular symptoms.
- Death is rarely the result of cardiovascular disease.
- Death usually results from pneumonia.
- Atrophy of paraspinous muscles leads to kyphoscoliosis.
- Poor respiratory function is due to involvement of diaphragm & accessory muscles & scoliosis.
- May have pulmonary hypertension from chronic sleep apnea

HEMATOLOGIC
N/A

METABOLIC/NUTRITIONAL
N/A

GASTROINTESTINAL
N/A

NEUROPSYCHIATRIC
N/A

MYASTHENIA GRAVIS

KARL WILLMANN, MD
D. B. COURSIN, MD

OVERVIEW
- Myasthenia gravis (MG) is an autoimmune disease in which antibodies act against acetylcholine receptors at the neuro-muscular junction, which results in weakness & easily fatigable muscles. The disease is classified into several groups depending on severity & muscles involved.
  - Group I: Ocular muscles only (20% of pts)
  - Group II A: Mild generalized symptoms, usually sparing respiratory muscles
  - Group II B: More severe, rapid progression of symptoms, may involve respiratory muscles
  - Group III: Rapid onset & progression, high mortality rate
  - Group IV: Severe form that usually is a progression of types IIA & IIB
- Incidence around 1 in 20,000; women affected twice as frequently as men
- 70–90% of patients w/ MG have circulating anti-acetylcholine receptor antibodies.
- T-helper cell activation in thymus leads to antibody formation.

- Antibodies damage postsynaptic membrane via complement-mediated reaction w/ increased degradation & decreased formation of acetylcholine receptors.
- 90% of pts have thymic abnormalities (atrophy, hyperplasia, thymoma).
- Poor correlation btwn levels of antibodies & clinical severity of disease.
- Associated often w/ other autoimmune diseases (systemic lupus erythematosus, rheumatoid arthritis, pernicious anemia, thyroiditis)
- May be initiated/exacerbated by viral infections, pregnancy, stress, surgery, hyperthermia
- Diagnosed by EMG, edrophonium test & presence of anti-acetylcholine receptor antibodies
- Therapeutic modalities include cholinesterase inhibitors (increase concentration of Ach at nicotinic postsynaptic membrane), thymectomy, immunosuppressants, corticosteroids, plasmapheresis.
- Pts often are taking anticholinesterases & immunosuppressive therapies, which will affect perioperative mgt.
- Underdosage of anticholinesterases can lead to skeletal muscle weakness.
- Overdosage of anticholinesterases can lead to abdominal cramping, vomiting, diarrhea, salivation, bradycardia, skeletal muscle weakness.

FLUID AND ELECTROLYTES
- Not significant except w/ renal failure related to meds

CARDIOPULMONARY
- Usually not significant
- Patients with both a thymoma & MG may have a focal myocarditis presenting as atrial fibrillation or atrioventricular block.

- Some association w/ LV diastolic dysfunction (but preservation of systolic function)
- In late stages, MG can precipitate significant respiratory failure.

HEMATOLOGIC
- Not significant except in relation to steroids & immunosuppressive meds

METABOLIC-NUTRITIONAL
- Not significant except if bulbar dysfunction makes adequate nutritional intake impossible

GASTROINTESTINAL
- No significant concerns

NEUROPSYCHIATRIC
- Skeletal muscle weakness, esp. w/ repetition
- May follow relapsing-remitting course
- Any muscle may be affected, although more likely to be innervated by cranial nerves
- Dysphagia, dysarthria, pulmonary aspiration, diplopia, lower limb weakness
- Consider MG in the differential diagnosis when assessing respiratory failure.

NEUROLEPTIC MALIGNANT SYNDROME

HUGH R. PLAYFORD, MD

OVERVIEW
N/A

FLUIDS AND ELECTROLYTES
- Acute phase
  - ➤ Hyperkalemia & renal insufficiency related to rhabdomyolysis

➤ Hypovolemia related to diaphoresis
■ Chronic
➤ Usually fully resolved

CARDIOPULMONARY
■ Acute phase
➤ May have signs of autonomic dysfunction (hypertension & hypotension, tachycardia, tachypnea, diaphoresis)
➤ Muscular weakness & rigidity may contribute to hypercapnic respiratory failure, failure of airway protective reflexes.
■ Chronic
➤ Usually fully resolved

HEMATOLOGIC
■ Acute
➤ Leukocytosis common
■ Chronic
➤ Usually fully resolved

METABOLIC-NUTRITIONAL
■ Not affected

GASTROINTESTINAL
■ Not affected

NEUROPSYCHIATRIC
■ Probably related to inhibition of central dopaminergic neurons by neuroleptic drugs
■ Typically associated w/ haloperidol, fluphenazine, clozapine, thiothixene, trifluoroperazine, thioridazine, chlorpromazine
■ Less commonly associated w/ droperidol, prochlorperazine, promethazine, metoclopramide
■ Also in Parkinson's pts w/ withdrawal of L-dopa
■ Variable relation to neuroleptic drugs (first day of therapy to after many months of therapy)
■ NOT ASSOCIATED W/ MALIGNANT HYPERTHERMIA

- No genetic association
- Clinical state
  - Hyperthermia
  - Muscle rigidity & weakness (may develop rhabdomyolysis & subsequent renal dysfunction)
  - Autonomic dysfunction (hypertension & hypotension, tachycardia, tachypnea, diaphoresis, urinary incontinence)
  - Mental status changes (delirium, mutism, stupor)
- Chronic sequelae may develop
  - Renal insufficiency/failure
  - Dementia, parkinsonism, cerebellar dysfunction
- Mgt largely supportive
  - Cessation of neuroleptic
  - Consider dantrolene, bromocriptine, L-dopa
  - ECT has been used in selected cases.
- Always consider the underlying reason for the use of neuroleptics in the first place!

OBSTETRIC PATIENT HAVING INTERCURRENT SURGERY

JONATHAN T. KETZLER, MD

OVERVIEW
- 2% of parturients have intercurrent surgery.
- 75,000 anesthetics per year
- Most commonly treated problems of this age group
  - Trauma
  - Appendicitis, cholelithiasis, torsion or ruptured ovarian cyst
  - Breast tumors
  - Cervical incompetence
- Less common but serious: intracranial aneurysms, cardiac valvular disease, pheochromocytoma

- Many are laparoscopic procedures.
- Preterm delivery is the greatest cause of fetal loss.
- Prevention & treatment of preterm labor is the most difficult problem to deal with.
  - ➤ Usually not related to anesthetic but rather to underlying disease & surgery
- Physiologic changes of pregnancy persist for 6 wks postpartum.
- Balance benefits of procedure against risks to both mother & child.
- Greatest risk of fetal death if procedure done in first trimester

FLUID & ELECTROLYTES
- Increased mineralocorticoid activity
  - ➤ Sodium retention
  - ➤ Increased body water content

CARDIOPULMONARY
- Cardiovascular
  - ➤ Increased cardiac output (up to 50%) secondary to increases in heart rate (15–20%) & stroke volume
  - ➤ Decrease in systemic (particularly in uterine & renal beds) & pulmonary vascular resistance
  - ➤ Decrease in vascular responsiveness, increase in baroreceptor responsiveness
  - ➤ Slight decrease in arterial pressure as vasodilatation exceeds increased CO
  - ➤ Aortocaval compression when supine unless positioned for left lateral uterine displacement
  - ➤ ECG may show left axis deviation, sinus tachycardia, premature atrial contractions, paroxysmal supraventricular tachycardia.
- Pulmonary
  - ➤ Higher oxygen consumption, lower pCO_2 due to elevated minute ventilation

- ➤ Decreased ERV, FRC, RV
- ➤ Increased IRV
- ➤ Thus, TLC remains the same.
- ➤ Increased mucosal vascularity (possible upper airway obstruction)
- ➤ Bronchorelaxation (secondary to progesterone)
- ➤ Lung compliance unchanged

HEMATOLOGIC
- ▪ Increases in total blood volume, plasma volume (both up to 40–50%)
- ▪ Increase in total red cell volume (20%)
- ▪ Dilutional anemia as increase in blood volume >increase in red cell mass
- ▪ Hb to 11–12 g/dL, Hct to 35%
- ▪ WBC to 8,000–10,000/mm^3
- ▪ Platelets generally unchanged
- ▪ Plasma fibrinogen increases by around 50%.
- ▪ Clotting factor activity variable
- ▪ Serum cholinesterase decreases by 20%.
- ▪ Decreased plasma proteins (albumin >globulins) may increase free concentration of protein-bound drugs.

METABOLIC/NUTRITIONAL
- ▪ Increased oxygen consumption (20% above normal)
- ▪ Hyperglycemia w/ glucose intolerance

GASTROINTESTINAL
- ▪ Gastric motility, pH & lower esophageal tone may be decreased.
- ▪ A parturient is considered a full stomach if she has eaten since her last menstrual period!

NEUROPSYCHIATRIC
- ▪ Requirement for local anesthetic decreased
- ▪ MAC for inhaled agents decreased

PARKINSON'S DISEASE

ROBERT N. SLADEN, MD

OVERVIEW
- Onset in sixth & seventh decade; family history; affects males >females
- Progressive necrosis of substantia nigra & CNS dopamine depletion
- Exacerbations & remissions
- Characteristic features
  - Tremor (forefinger & thumb, "pill rolling")
  - Rigidity (+ tremor = "cogwheel rigidity")
  - Bradykinesia (loss of facial expression, slurring of speech)
  - Increased secretions
- Systemic disease w/ generalized debility
  - Anemia
  - Muscle wasting
  - Poor nutrition
  - Susceptible to aspiration, infection, hypothermia

FLUID & ELECTROLYTES
N/A

CARDIOPULMONARY
- Chronic dopaminergic therapy
  - Vasodilation, systemic hypotension

HEMATOLOGIC
N/A

METABOLIC/NUTRITIONAL
N/A

GASTROINTESTINAL
N/A

NEUROPSYCHIATRIC
- Tremor, rigidity, bradykinesia (see above)
- Intellectual function preserved

PATIENT WITH A TRANSPLANT

ARTHUR ATCHABAHIAN, MD

OVERVIEW

Immunosuppression
- Corticosteroids
- Cyclosporine (Neoral or Sandimmune), FK-506 (tacrolimus, Prograf)
  - Both meds target T-lymphocytes.
  - Nephrotoxicity through renal vasoconstriction (cyclosporine >FK-506)
  - Hypertension, hyperkalemia, hyperglycemia
  - Neurotoxicity (tremors, confusion, seizures)
- Rapamycin (sirolimus, Rapamune)
  - Targets T cells through a mechanism different from cyclosporine & FK-506
  - Thrombocytopenia, dyslipidemia
- Mycophenolate (Cellcept), azathioprine (Imuran)
  - Antimetabolites that inhibit lymphocyte proliferation
  - Leukopenia, thrombocytopenia, anemia
- Monoclonal antibodies (only IV, administered to treat acute rejection)
  - Possible severe pulmonary edema w/ OKT-3

Other meds
- Prophylactic antibiotics
  - TMP-SMX to prevent PCP (usually long-term)
  - Ganciclovir or acyclovir to prevent CMV & EBV (usually only during periods of intense immunosuppression)

Indication for transplant

- Heart Tx: CAD, dilated CM, viral myocarditis
- Renal Tx: diabetes mellitus, vasculitis, glomerulonephritis, uncontrolled hypertension, obstruction
- Liver Tx: cirrhosis w/ or w/out potential for recurrence, biliary malformation, acute hepatic failure
- Lung Tx: cystic fibrosis, end-stage emphysema, alpha-1 antitrypsin deficiency, primary pulmonary hypertension
- Time elapsed since transplantation (determines risk of rejection & susceptibility to infection)

Transplant function

- History of rejection (2 episodes of rejection on average for heart Tx recipients)

FLUIDS AND ELECTROLYTES

- Steroid treatment w/ possible water & sodium retention
- Chronic renal insufficiency possible because of renal toxicity of some immunosuppressants, esp. cyclosporine
- Hepatorenal syndrome associated w/ chronic liver dysfunction
- Osteoporosis is a side effect of long-standing steroid treatment.

CARDIOPULMONARY

Evaluate for CAD

- Pts often at risk because of diabetes mellitus, hypercholesterolemia, hypertension, smoking history

Heart Tx

- Denervated w/ no vagal inflow
  - ➤ Resting heart rate increased
  - ➤ No response to anticholinergics such as atropine
  - ➤ Normal response to circulating catecholamines
- Susceptible to accelerated atherosclerosis

> Typically diffuse lesions not accessible to angioplasty or revascularization
- Frank-Starling mechanism is the main mechanism to adjust cardiac output
  > Maintain adequate fluid status to preserve preload
- A portion of the native atria remains
  > Possibly two types of P waves on EKG

Liver Tx
- If cirrhotic, peripheral & pulmonary shunting may take time to normalize.
- Pleural effusion possible, especially on the right side
- Ascites may decrease FRC.

Renal Tx
- Hyperdynamic circulation with fixed low SVR & peripheral shunting may take time to normalize.

Lung Tx
- Loss of ciliary function because of denervation
  > Propensity to mucous plugging & pneumonia
- Single lung: contralateral diseased lung still present, w/ shunt

HEMATOLOGIC
- Anemia due to malnutrition, bone marrow suppression by immunosuppressive treatment, frequent blood sampling
- Thrombocytopenia due to bone marrow suppression
- Leukopenia due to bone marrow suppression
- Coagulopathy due to uremia, hepatic insufficiency

METABOLIC-NUTRITIONAL
- Induced glucose intolerance or diabetes mellitus, preexisting or secondary to steroid treatment
- Malnutrition
- Hypercatabolism due to steroid treatment

GASTROINTESTINAL
- Gl bleed due to steriods, uremia, esophageal varices

NEUROPSYCHIATRIC

- ■ Possible neuropsychiatric side effects of immunosuppressive treatment
  - ➤ Confusion, seizures, coma
- ■ Sensory and/or autonomic neuropathy due to diabetes mellitus and/or uremia

---

PHEOCHROMOCYTOMA

GIUDITTA ANGELINI, MD

OVERVIEW

- ■ Adrenal medulla tumors produce, store & secrete catecholamines (both epinephrine & norepinephrine).
- ■ Occur in 0.1% of hypertensive pts
- ■ Undiagnosed & untreated, there is a high mortality.
- ■ Surgical management curative in around 90%
- ■ Present in third to fifth decade of life in both genders w/ hypertension (sometimes paroxysmal w/ heart failure, MI, dysrhythmias, cerebral hemorrhage), headache, palpitations, tremor, diaphoresis, pallor or flushing
- ■ 5% inherited as autosomal dominant
- ■ May be part of MEN IIA or IIB
- ■ 10% multiple tumors, 10% extra-adrenal, 10% malignant
- ■ Differential diagnosis includes:
  - ➤ Essential hypertension
    - Unknown cause
  - ➤ Primary renal disease
    - Nephritis, renal artery stenosis, renal infarction
  - ➤ Endocrine
    - Adrenocortical hyperfunction, thyroid disease, pheochromocytoma, acromegaly
  - ➤ Hemodynamic alterations
    - Increased peripheral resistance, increased intravascular volume

- ➤ Sympathetic stimulation
  - Light anesthesia, hypoxia, hypercarbia
- ➤ Neurogenic
  - Seizure activity, elevated ICP, denervation of carotid sinus
- ➤ Miscellaneous
  - Malignant hyperthermia, neuroleptic malignant syndrome, carcinoid syndrome, toxemia of pregnancy

FLUID AND ELECTROLYTES

- Pts w/ pheochromocytoma may have elevated blood sugar.
- Reduced intravascular volume

CARDIOPULMONARY

- Sympathetic paraganglia are a possible location for a pheochromocytoma.
- Epinephrine, norepinephrine, dopamine are usually secreted from the tumor.
- Beta-adrenergic stimulation
  - ➤ Adenylcyclase stimulates production of cAMP & subsequent inward Ca++ flux w/ enhanced myosin & actin interactions.
- Alpha-adrenergic stimulation
  - ➤ Enhances Ca++ influx as well but also inositol triphosphate
- Synthesis of catecholamines
  - ➤ Active transport of tyrosine into postganglionic sympathetic nerve endings
- Breakdown by catechol-o-methyl transferase (COMT)
- Also breakdown by monoamine oxidase (MAO)
- Diaphoresis & palpitations are common associated symptoms of pheochromocytoma.
- Hypertension can be paroxysmal in 35%; otherwise sustained
- Left ventricular hypertrophy clinically & on ECG
- Catecholamine-induced cardiomyopathy may present as heart failure and/or dysrhythmias.

■ Chest x-ray may show cardiomegaly.

HEMATOLOGIC

■ Hemoconcentration secondary to reduced intravascular volume

METABOLIC-NUTRITIONAL

■ Weight loss, pallor & fever can all be symptoms of pheochromocytoma.

GASTROINTESTINAL

■ Most often found in the adrenal medulla
■ Symptoms of pheochromocytoma can include nausea & vomiting.

NEUROPSYCHIATRIC

■ Found in the chromaffin cells of the sympathetic nervous system
■ Headache is a common symptom of pheochromocytoma.
■ Pts can become encephalopathic from hypertension.

PLATELET DISORDERS

KARL WILLMANN, MD

OVERVIEW

■ There are numerous platelet disorders, w/ many etiologies.
■ Abnormalities of platelet number or platelet function
■ Thrombocytopenia
  ➤ Platelet dilution
  ➤ Platelet destruction
  ➤ Platelet consumption
  ➤ Inadequate platelet production
  ➤ Sequestration
■ Decreased function

➤ Uremia
➤ Antiplatelet agents (cyclooxygenase agents, PDEi, adenosine receptor antagonists, glycoprotein IIb/IIIa receptor antagonists, cephalosporins & some penicillins)

■ Drugs, viral illness, massive transfusion, renal disease, autoimmune disease, excessive destruction or sequestration, decreased production, congenital, preeclampsia, HELLP syndrome & idiopathic causes are often the source of platelet dysfunction & decreased number, which lead to a bleeding diathesis.

■ Heparin-induced thrombocytopenia (HIT) may develop in up to 5% of patients who receive heparin.
➤ Development of thrombocytopenia variable in onset
➤ May present as thrombocytopenia, bleeding, thrombosis
➤ IgG antibodies directed against platelet-heparin complexes

FLUID AND ELECTROLYTES
■ No special concerns

CARDIOPULMONARY
■ No special concerns

HEMATOLOGIC
■ Massive transfusions can lead to a dilutional thrombocytopenia.
■ Cardiac bypass can lead to platelet destruction & thrombocytopenia.
■ Disease processes such as myeloproliferative & dysplastic syndromes may produce low numbers & dysfunctional platelets.
■ Bone marrow suppression related to radiation & chemotherapy may lead to thrombocytopenia.
■ In DIC there may an accelerated use of platelets, leading to a decreased platelet count.

- Other autoimmune diseases may lead to platelet destruction, such as rheumatoid arthritis, thrombocytopenia purpura, systemic lupus erythematosus.
- There may be splenic sequestration of platelets, leading to thrombocytopenia.

METABOLIC-NUTRITIONAL
- No special concerns

GASTROINTESTINAL
- H_2 blocking drugs such as cimetidine & ranitidine may have a deleterious effect on platelet production/destruction.
- Hepatic failure may contribute to thrombocytopenia via bone marrow suppression.
- Uremia may lead to poor platelet function related to toxic compounds that decrease the ability of platelets to bind to exposed endothelium.
- These compounds can be dialyzed off; therefore, dialysis can improve platelet function.
- There may also be some interaction w/ von Willebrand factor, causing poor platelet function. This may respond to desmopressin (DDAVP) therapy.
- Renal failure may also affect bone marrow production of platelets.

NEUROPSYCHIATRIC
- No special concerns

POLYCYTHEMIA

KARL WILLMANN, MD, AND DOUGLAS B. COURSIN, MD

OVERVIEW
- Polycythemia is defined as abnormally high Hgb (>16.5 in women or >18.5 in men) or Hct (>48 in women or >52 in men) due to increased number of RBCs.

- Polycythemia classified as:
  - Relative: an increase in Hct or Hgb due to a decrease in plasma volume
    - Occurs w/ dehydration
    - May be a chronic process (obesity, hypertension, other)
  - Absolute: absolute real increase in red cell mass, also known as erythrocytosis
  - Primary
    - Inherited or acquired mutation that results in abnormal erythroid production
      - Most common cause is polycythemia vera
        - A myeloproliferative process (includes CML, essential thrombocytopenia, myeloid metaplasia) that results in an increase in all cell lines, RBCs, platelets & white cells
        - Slightly more common in men, usually over 50
        - Starts as a latent & relatively asymptomatic process, then converts to a proliferative phase where pts are increasingly at risk for hyperviscosity
          - Pts frequently have headaches, diastolic hypertension, plethora, injected conjunctiva.
          - May complain of periodic burning in fingers & toes from ischemia
          - Hepatosplenomegaly from proliferation
        - Platelets are dysfunctional.
      - More rarely, a familial variant
  - Secondary
    - Caused by circulating plasma factors that stimulate erythropoiesis
      - Most commonly erythropoietin (EPO)
        - Seen pathologically in tumors that secrete EPO (endocrine, liver, uterine, renal)
      - Occurs in smokers, hypoxemic pts, those living at altitude, morbidly obese, COPD, obstructive sleep apnea

- Heavy smokers (>1 ppd) have increased carboxyhemoglobin levels w/ a very high affinity for oxygen; may result in poor oxygen delivery to tissues, causing hypoxia.
  - Hct usually <55%
➤ Unapparent polycythemia: red cell mass is increased, but so is the plasma volume, so polycythemia is unrecognized
➤ Most commonly secondary to chronic hypoxia or an EPO-secreting renal tumor, less commonly polycythemia vera
➤ Differentiate etiology by history, physical, lab testing.
  - History: smoker, chronic lung disease, carbon monoxide exposure, blood doping w/ EPO, gout, family history, pruritus, vascular effects (TIAs, angina, peripheral vascular thrombosis), bleeding, peptic ulceration, abdominal discomfort from nephrolithiasis or splenomegaly
  - Physical exam: SpO_2, cyanosis, clubbing, hepatosplenomegaly, breathing pattern
  - Labs
    - Polycythemia vera
      - High WBCs, platelets
      - High Hgb, Hct
      - Low plasma volume
      - Sat > 92% on room air unless underlying pulmonary pathology, CO level < 5%
      - Low serum EPO level in polycythemia vera
      - May also see increased bilirubin, uric acid
➤ Main one we need to be concerned about is polycythemia vera, because of associated risk of thrombosis, bleeding & increased perioperative morbidity & mortality if unrecognized & untreated.
  - Initial treatment: lower Hct via phlebotomy to <46%
  - Bleeding & thrombosis (arterial and/or venous) are the major complications.

FLUID AND ELECTROLYTES
- Maintain normovolemia to limit sludging & potential for thrombosis. See "Hematologic" section.
- Pts may have hyperuricemia w/ increased risk for gout or kidney stones.

CARDIOPULMONARY
- Increased risk for myocardial ischemia when Hct very high & w/ abnormal prothrombotic platelet dysfunction; see "Hematologic" section

HEMATOLOGIC
- The most significant risk is for both arterial & venous thrombosis.
  - Increased viscosity w/ higher Hct
  - Increased thrombosis from platelet dysfunction as well as increased risk for bleeding
  - Pts at risk for myocardial ischemia/infarction, cerebral ischemia/stroke, peripheral arterial occlusion, deep vein thrombosis
- Therapy for polycythemia may induce AML (radioactive phosphate, busulphan).

METABOLIC-NUTRITIONAL
- Due to the increased production of red blood cells, pts may be iron-deficient.

GASTROINTESTINAL
- Pts w/ hepatic vein thrombosis may be at increased risk for gastric and esophageal varices & bleeding as well as liver dysfunction.
- Patients may have hyperuricemia with increased risk for gout or kidney stones.

NEUROPSYCHIATRIC
- No specific considerations

PSYCHIATRIC DISORDERS

JONATHAN T. KETZLER, MD

OVERVIEW

- Depression
  - ➤ Mood disorder characterized by sadness & pessimism
  - ➤ Usually multifactorial in origin
  - ➤ Treatment is based on the presumption that manifestations are due to brain deficiency of dopamine, norepinephrine & serotonin or due to altered receptor activities.
  - ➤ As many as 50% of pts w/ severe depression have high levels of cortisol.
- Mania
  - ➤ Mood disorder characterized by elation, hyperactivity & flight of ideas
  - ➤ May alternate w/ depression
  - ➤ Thought to be due to high levels of norepinephrine in the brain
  - ➤ Treated primarily w/ lithium but may add haloperidol or lorazepam
- Schizophrenia
  - ➤ Pt displays disordered thinking, withdrawal, paranoid delusions & auditory hallucinations.
  - ➤ Thought to be due to excess levels of dopamine in the brain
  - ➤ Antipsychotic drugs are the only treatment.
- Neuroleptic malignant syndrome (NMS)
  - ➤ A rare complication of antipsychotic therapy
  - ➤ Haloperidol most common inducing agent but also associated w/ butyrophenones, phenothiazines & thioxanthenes
  - ➤ Occurs hrs to wks after administration
  - ➤ Manifest by muscle rigidity, hyperthermia, rhabdomyolysis, autonomic instability & altered consciousness

- ➤ Fatal in 20–30% of cases; death caused by renal failure or dysrhythmias
- ➤ Treated w/ dantrolene or bromocriptine
- ➤ Pts w/ history of NMS should be treated the same as pts w/ potential for malignant hyperthermia.

FLUID & ELECTROLYTES
N/A

CARDIOPULMONARY
N/A

HEMATOLOGIC
N/A

METABOLIC/NUTRITIONAL
N/A

GASTROINTESTINAL
N/A

NEUROPSYCHIATRIC
N/A

RESTRICTIVE LUNG DISEASE

HUGH R. PLAYFORD, MBBS

OVERVIEW
- ■ Extrapulmonary abnormalities
  - ➤ Abdomen: obesity, pregnancy, ascites
  - ➤ Skin: circumferential skin burns w/ contractures, obesity
  - ➤ Musculoskeletal: kyphoscoliosis (combination of kyphosis & scoliosis), scoliosis alone, kyphosis alone, thoracoplasty, syringomyelia, vertebral & spinal cord tumors, poliomyelitis
  - ➤ Pleural: pleural effusion, empyema
- ■ Pulmonary interstitial abnormalities

➤ Idiopathic pulmonary fibrosis (IPF)/cryptogenic fibrosis alveolitis (CFA) most common (3–8/100,000 persons)

➤ Other causes include the fibroproliferative phase of acute respiratory distress syndrome (ARDS), desquamative interstitial pneumonia (DIP), respiratory bronchiolitis interstitial lung disease (RBILD), nonspecific interstitial pneumonia (NSIP), acute interstitial pneumonia (AIP), lymphoid interstitial pneumonia (LIP), cryptogenic organizing pneumonia.

FLUIDS AND ELECTROLYTES
■ Usually normal

CARDIOPULMONARY
■ Usually progresses toward respiratory failure
  ➤ IPF
    • Progressive course w/out spontaneous remissions irrespective of therapy
    • Respiratory failure within 3–8 yrs of onset of symptoms
    • Subset of pts stabilize after an initial period of decline.
    • Mean survival of IPF from the onset of symptoms is about 3–5 yrs.
  ➤ Kyphoscoliosis
    • More indolent course
    • Clinical symptoms correlate to the degree of the spinal curvature.
    • Some pts remain asymptomatic; others progress to respiratory failure & cor pulmonale.
    • Pts w/ scoliotic curve of >70 degrees are at high risk of developing respiratory failure.
    • Spinal curvature tends to increase with age by about 15 degrees every 20 yrs.
    • Angles >100 degrees are associated w/ dyspnea; >120 degrees may result in alveolar hypoventilation & cor pulmonale.

- ➤ Cor pulmonale from hypoxemic pulmonary vasoconstriction or anatomic abnormalities; may be treated by supplemental oxygen, correction of reversible causes of hypercapnia, mgt of sleep-disordered breathing
- ➤ Initial symptoms are cough (usually nonproductive) & dyspnea.
  - Cough may become paroxysmal & debilitating.
  - Fevers, sweats, chills suggest intercurrent infection.
- ➤ Late phases develop cyanosis & cor pulmonale.
- ➤ Examination
  - Rapid, shallow breathing pattern
  - End-inspiratory rales ("Velcro"-like) in around 85%
  - Clubbing present in 25–93%, hypertrophic osteo-arthropathy
  - May have evidence of pulmonary hypertension (loud P_2, right ventricular heave, jugular venous distention), right ventricular failure (dependent edema, hepatomegaly)
- ◼ PFTs
  - ➤ PFT abnormalities correlate poorly w/ the angle of the deformity.
  - ➤ Relate to loss of normal thoracic kyphosis, location of the curve, number of vertebral bodies involved
  - ➤ ↓ TLC, ↓ VC, ↓ IC (TLC-FRC), ↓ FRC
  - ➤ ↓ or normal RV, ↓ ERV (FRC-RV)
  - ➤ ↓ FEV_1
  - ➤ ↓ Diffusing capacity (V/Q inequality & ↓ vascular bed)
  - ➤ Alveolar hypoventilation from ↑ V_D/V_T ratio
  - ➤ ↓V_T w/ preservation of anatomic & alveolar dead space
  - ➤ ↓V_T allows a decreased work of breathing.
  - ➤ ↓ Pulmonary compliance
  - ➤ Pressure-volume curves are shifted downward & to the right.
- ◼ ABGs
  - ➤ Kyphoscoliosis

- Usually normal oxygenation until pt develops hypercapnia
- Nocturnal hypoxemia & hypercapnia may develop earlier.
- AAG usually <25 mm Hg, even in late stages (V/Q inequality, underventilation of hemithorax)
➤ IPF
  - Resting hypoxemia
  - Mild respiratory alkalosis

HEMATOLOGIC
- Polycythemia may be present secondary to chronic polycythemia.

METABOLIC-NUTRITIONAL
- High work of breathing increases metabolic load, elevates resting energy expenditure.
- Malnutrition may be present.

GASTROINTESTINAL
- Not significantly involved

NEUROPSYCHIATRIC
- Not significantly involved

RHEUMATOID ARTHRITIS

ROBERT N. SLADEN, MD

OVERVIEW
- Systemic disease w/ generalized debility
  ➤ Anemia
  ➤ Muscle wasting
  ➤ Poor nutrition
  ➤ Susceptible to infection, hypothermia
- Progressive bilateral, symmetrical arthropathy

➤ Knees, elbows, wrists, metacarpophalangeal, metatar-
sophalangeal
➤ Impaired mobility
➤ Severe deformity: difficult positioning & access
■ Airway considerations
➤ Temporomandibular joint (limited mouth opening)
➤ Atlantoaxial joint, odontoid process (limited head exten-
sion, flexion)

FLUID & ELECTROLYTES
N/A

CARDIOPULMONARY
■ Restrictive lung disease
➤ Rheumatoid nodules
➤ Interstitial pulmonary fibrosis
■ Pleural effusions

HEMATOLOGIC
N/A

METABOLIC/NUTRITIONAL
N/A

GASTROINTESTINAL
N/A

NEUROPSYCHIATRIC
N/A

SCLERODERMA

ARTHUR ATCHABAHIAN, MD

OVERVIEW
■ New name is "systemic sclerosis."
■ Pathogenesis is related to small vessel destruction & fibrosis
of skin & multiple organs

- ➤ Widespread symmetric, leathery induration of skin
- ➤ Involvement of muscles, bones, heart, lungs, intestinal tract
- CREST syndrome: calcinosis, Raynaud's phenomenon, esophageal hypomotility, sclerodactyly, telangiectasis
  - ➤ This variant is usually more benign & less progressive.
- A variety of autoantibodies are found in scleroderma, including antibodies to smooth muscle, rheumatoid factor, antinuclear antibodies (ANA) & antibodies to nuclear components.
  - ➤ ANA & antibodies to Scl-70 (a non-histone nuclear protein) are highly specific for scleroderma.
  - ➤ Antibodies to centromere are associated w/ CREST syndrome.
- More common in women 30–50 yrs of age
- Pregnancy can accelerate progression of disease; high incidence of spontaneous abortion & premature labor
- Acute renal failure is the leading cause of death.
- Musculoskeletal
  - ➤ Thickening & non-pitting edema of skin
    - Later on, skin becomes tight, w/ flexion contractures.
  - ➤ Proximal myopathy w/ elevated CK
  - ➤ Inflammatory arthritis, possible avascular necrosis of femoral head
  - ➤ Nonerosive synovitis leading to carpal tunnel syndrome

FLUIDS AND ELECTROLYTES

- Possible involvement of renal arteries w/ progression to renal failure
  - ➤ Acute drop in renal blood flow can trigger acute renal failure w/ malignant hypertension, a medical emergency.
  - ➤ Symptoms include headache, visual disturbances, encephalopathy, seizures, oligo-anuria, edema, CHF, arrhythmias.
  - ➤ Physiopathology is hyperreninemia due to renal angiopathy, leading to severe renal vasospasm.

➤ Treatment of acute renal crisis w/ ACE inhibitors has significantly reduced mortality.

➤ Treatment of malignant hypertension w/ sodium nitroprusside or nicardipine is necessary in addition to ACE inhibitor administration.

➤ Normotensive renal crisis is possible, especially in pts receiving high doses of steroids.

■ Pt may be on steroid therapy, w/ associated side effects.

CARDIOPULMONARY

■ Rare myocardial fibrosis leading to CHF; more common if myositis

■ Dysrhythmias or conduction abnormalities

■ Pericarditis, pericardial effusion, w/ or w/out tamponade

■ Oral & nasal telangiectasias

■ Hypertension from involvement of renal arteries

■ CREST syndrome

■ Near-constant pulmonary restrictive syndrome & impaired diffusion capacity from fibrosis, similar to idiopathic pulmonary fibrosis

■ Common thickening of pulmonary vessels w/ pulmonary hypertension leading to cor pulmonale

■ Increase in dead space from widening of airways

HEMATOLOGIC

■ Possible impaired coagulation due to malabsorption of vitamin K from intestinal hypomotility & bacterial overgrowth

METABOLIC-NUTRITIONAL

■ Pt may be on steroid therapy, with associated side effects.

■ Possible malabsorption from intestinal hypomotility & bacterial overgrowth

GASTROINTESTINAL

■ Oral dryness

■ Esophageal hypomotility & reduced lower esophageal sphincter tone

- Bacterial overgrowth from intestinal hypomotility

NEUROPSYCHIATRIC

- Cranial nerve neuropathy because of compression by thickened connective tissue
- Dry keratoconjunctivitis

SICKLE CELL DISEASE

ARTHUR ATCHABAHIAN, MD

OVERVIEW

- Abnormal beta chain of hemoglobin due to substitution of valine for glutamic acid at the 6 position. The abnormal hemoglobin is designated HbS.
- Sickle cell trait (heterozygous): 10% black population in the US; 20–40% HbS. Asymptomatic.
- Sickle cell disease (homozygous): 0.3–1% black population in the US; 70–98% HbS. Anemia with Hb 5–10 g/dL. Survival beyond age 30 is rare.
- Diagnosis by electrophoresis of Hb
- HbS tends to form aggregates (*tactoids*) when deoxygenated, hence sickling of erythrocytes, with shortened life span (10–20 days instead of 120).
  - ➤ Oxyhemoglobin dissociation curve also shifted to the right
    - Increased intracellular 2,3 DPG; facilitates oxygen delivery to tissues
  - ➤ Homozygous: sickling at tissue PO_2 of 40 mm Hg
  - ➤ Heterozygous: sickling at tissue PO_2 of 20 mm Hg
  - ➤ Sickling also triggered by
    - Acidosis
    - Hypothermia
    - Dehydration
    - Blood stasis

- ➤ Radiographic contrast dye causes sickling in vitro.
    - Risks of angiography are unclear.
- ➤ Vaso-occlusion is more likely w/ a higher Hct
    - Predicted final Hct is a criterion for choosing btwn transfusion & exchange transfusion.
    - Keep Hct around 25–30.
- ■ Acute complications
    - ➤ Vaso-occlusive crisis
    - ➤ Chest syndrome
    - ➤ Hepatic crisis
    - ➤ Bone marrow necrosis & fat embolism
    - ➤ Cerebral vascular occlusion
    - ➤ Priapism
    - ➤ Splenic infarction & sequestration
    - ➤ Aplastic crisis
    - ➤ Asplenic sepsis syndrome
- ■ Musculoskeletal
    - ➤ Common avascular femoral head necrosis
    - ➤ Rare bone marrow necrosis w/ fat embolism
        - Fever, severe bone pain, neurologic signs & respiratory distress
        - Exchange transfusion can be lifesaving.
    - ➤ Osteomyelitis, often caused by *Salmonella* sp.
    - ➤ Gout common because of the increased nucleic acid catabolism
    - ➤ Leg ulcers common

FLUIDS AND ELECTROLYTES

- ■ Renal medulla site of frequent occlusive events because of low tissue PO_2
    - ➤ Papillary necrosis w/ hematuria
    - ➤ Impaired ability to concentrate urine
    - ➤ Leads to renal failure

- Even pts w/ sickle cell trait have been shown to develop medullary infarcts & to have a higher incidence of hematuria.

CARDIOPULMONARY

- High cardiac output due to anemia, w/ common flow murmur
- LV dysfunction can be a consequence of chronic transfusion w/ iron deposition.
- Cor pulmonale secondary to repeated pulmonary emboli
- Multiple pulmonary infarcts lead to increased A-a gradient, decreased TLC & FVC.
- Acute chest syndrome
  - ➤ Painful crisis
  - ➤ Fever
  - ➤ Pleuritic chest pain
  - ➤ Pulmonary infiltrate, often transient
  - ➤ Differential includes pneumonia & pulmonary embolism.
  - ➤ Supportive treatment w/ analgesics, hydration & oxygen therapy
  - ➤ Consider exchange transfusion if PO_2 cannot be maintained >75 mm Hg.

HEMATOLOGIC

- Splenomegaly frequent in small children
  - ➤ Because of repeated infarcts, most pts are functionally asplenic by age 6.
  - ➤ Decreased production of antibodies & increased risk of bacterial infection (esp. encapsulated organisms such as *Streptococcus pneumoniae* & *Haemophilus influenzae*; also *E. coli* UTI & *Salmonella* osteomyelitis)
  - ➤ Pts w/ less severe forms (eg, Hb SC disease) will still have a functional spleen into adulthood.
- Vaso-occlusive crisis
  - ➤ Often triggered by infection or trauma
  - ➤ Acute onset of intense pain, often abdominal or thoracic

- ➤ May last only minutes or as long as 3 wks
- ➤ Treat w/ analgesics, hydration, alkalinization & oxygen supplementation.
- ■ Aplastic crisis
  - ➤ Bone marrow depression triggered by viral infections (parvovirus B19)
  - ➤ Fever, anorexia, nausea & vomiting, headache, abdominal pain
  - ➤ Severe anemia w/ mild leukopenia & thrombocytopenia, low reticulocyte count
  - ➤ Self-limited, with recovery usually by 2 wks
  - ➤ Treat w/ transfusion as needed.
- ■ Sequestration crisis
  - ➤ Pooling of erythrocytes in spleen & liver
  - ➤ Left upper quadrant pain, shock
  - ➤ Possible acute hypovolemia or even sudden death
  - ➤ Immediate transfusion
- ■ Priapism
  - ➤ May resolve spontaneously w/ supportive treatment or necessitate exchange transfusion and/or surgery

METABOLIC-NUTRITIONAL
- ■ Usually normal

GASTROINTESTINAL
- ■ The liver is also a site of vascular occlusion
  - ➤ Painful enlargement
  - ➤ Hyperbilirubinemia
  - ➤ Function usually preserved
  - ➤ Decreased activity of plasma cholinesterase possible
- ■ Chronic hemolysis leads to elevated plasma bilirubin
  - ➤ High incidence of cholelithiasis
- ■ Chronic transfusion leads to a high prevalence of viral hepatitis
  - ➤ In some cases to iron overload w/ cirrhosis

NEUROPSYCHIATRIC
- Vascular occlusion manifests as cerebral infarcts in children & hemorrhage in adults
  - Treatment w/ exchange transfusion
  - Recurrence rate decreased by maintenance transfusions

SPINAL CORD INJURY

HUGH R. PLAYFORD, MBBS, AND GEBHARD WAGENER, MD

OVERVIEW
- Acute: Spinal shock

Definition
- Up to 3 wks after injury
- Loss of sensation, temperature regulation & spinal cord reflexes below injury
- Mortality due to
  - Aspiration
  - Respiratory failure
  - Pneumonia

Chronic stage
- >3 wks after injury
  - Sympathetic system hyperactive: autonomic hyper-reflexia
  - Spinal reflexes return
  - Chronic infections: urinary tract, pulmonary
  - Renal failure often causes significant mortality.
  - Transection above C2 to C4 causes paralysis of the diaphragm.
  - Pt cannot maintain adequate oxygenation & ventilation, requiring immediate intubation & mechanical ventilation.
  - Musculoskeletal
    - *Acute:*

- Flaccidity below injury
- *Chronic:*
  - Osteoporosis, muscular atrophy & pathologic fractures common
  - Muscle spasm & spasticity requiring medication
  - Contractures requiring intense physiotherapy and/or surgery
  - Decubital ulcers common

FLUIDS AND ELECTROLYTES

- Acute
  - Pt may have significant intravascular volume depletion, depending on other injuries & degree of systemic vasodilatation.
  - Hyponatremia common in acute stages
- Chronic
  - Hypercalcemia from prolonged immobilization
  - Renal insufficiency common (chronic urinary tract infections, nephrolithiasis)

CARDIOPULMONARY

- Acute
  - Altered autonomic outflow (initial hyperactivity, then hypoactivity)
  - Short-lived hypertension (increased systemic vascular resistance, increased cardiac contractility, increased dysrhythmias), then hypotension (decreased systemic vascular resistance w/ blood pooling in the capacitance vessels) & bradycardia (decreased activity of the T1-4 cardiac accelerator fibers) leading to spinal shock
  - Spinal shock typically lasts for 3 days to about 6 wks.
  - In the setting of unopposed vagal tone, the usual tachycardic response to hypovolemia & hypotension may not be seen.

- ➤ Cardiac arrest: occasionally seen on tracheal suctioning, esp. in the presence of hypoxia (unopposed vasovagal reflex)
- ➤ Cardiopulmonary changes may also be related to other injuries (thoracic, hemorrhage, etc.).
- ➤ Injuries above C5 lead to diaphragmatic paralysis (w/ paradoxical abdominal excursion); pt will need ventilatory support.
- ➤ Pts w/ injuries above T1 may have significant hypoventilation.
- ➤ Pulmonary edema related to neurogenic etiology (transient centrally mediated alpha-adrenergic sympathetic discharge) or excessive fluid replacement
- ➤ Beta2-agonist nebulizer therapy may further decrease SVR & contribute to hypotension.
- ➤ Pulmonary embolism: secondary to prolonged immobilization
- ■ Chronic
  - ➤ Pulmonary complications are very common, particularly w/ high cervical spine injuries.
  - ➤ Pts w/ injuries above T1 may have significant hypoventilation.
  - ➤ Injuries above C5 lead to diaphragmatic paralysis; pt will need ventilatory support.
  - ➤ Pulmonary function improves w/ intercostals & abdominal muscle spasticity leading to increased abdominal muscle elastic recoil & decreased end-expiratory volume.
  - ➤ Hypoventilation leads to V/Q inequality, increased dead space, hypoxia, hypercarbia, pulmonary vasoconstriction, sputum retention, atelectasis, pneumonia & respiratory failure.
  - ➤ PFTs: decreased VC, decreased TV, decreased TLC, decreased ERV, decreased FEV1, decreased FVC, decreased expiratory flow rates, decreased FRC, increased residual volume

- ➤ Postural hypotension & bradycardia (esp. if level above T4)
- ➤ ABGs may show hypoxemia w/ or w/out hypercarbia.
- ➤ Cardiac arrest: occasionally seen on tracheal suctioning, esp. in the presence of hypoxia (unopposed vasovagal reflex)
- ➤ Pulmonary embolism: secondary to prolonged immobilization

HEMATOLOGIC

- ■ Acute
  - ➤ Anemia is usually a consequence of other injuries & hemodilution (to manage hypotension related to systemic vasodilatation).
- ■ Chronic
  - ➤ Very high risk of DVTs, PTEs
  - ➤ Iatrogenic coagulopathy from prophylactic or therapeutic anticoagulants
  - ➤ Anemia from chronic renal insufficiency or chronic use of NSAIDs

METABOLIC-NUTRITIONAL

- ■ High injury level (above T1) may interfere w/ thermoregulation, leading to poikilothermia.

GASTROINTESTINAL

- ■ Acute
  - ➤ Gastric retention leading to gastric atony, paralytic ileus, abdominal distention
- ■ Chronic
  - ➤ High risk of constipation, needing long-term use of laxatives & purgatives
  - ➤ GI bleeding related to NSAIDs

NEUROPSYCHIATRIC

- ■ Incidence 11.5 to 53.4 per million population
- ■ Typically

➤ Males 15–25 yrs
➤ Related to motor vehicle accidents
➤ Involve cervical spine (often C5/6)
➤ Most common site of thoracolumbar injury is T12/L1.
■ Associated w/ other trauma in 25–65% of cases
➤ Consider spinal cord injury in all polytrauma or unconscious patients UNTIL PROVEN OTHERWISE!
➤ Head (including intracranial injury, facial injuries)
➤ Consider the possibility of vertebral artery injury (esp. if brain stem or cerebellar dysfunction).
➤ Thorax (rib fractures, hemothorax, pneumothorax)
■ Acute manifestations depend on the injury (primary & secondary; eg, hypotension & hypoxemia), level of injury, area of injury (complete or incomplete) & may give a pattern of spinal shock.
➤ Sensory: loss of visceral & somatic sensation
➤ Motor: flaccid paralysis, absent deep tendon reflexes, abdominal reflexes & plantar responses
➤ Autonomic: initial hypertension, then hypotension & bradycardia, retention of feces & urine, poikilothermia
➤ Psychological issues: frequent development of depression
■ Spinal cord blood flow influenced by:
➤ MAP (normal autoregulation 50–150 mm Hg, may be disrupted in injury)
➤ Arterial $PaCO_2$ (blood flow increases linearly from 50 to 90 mm Hg, decreases w/ hyperventilation)
➤ Endogenous endorphins (decrease blood flow by inducing hyperventilation & hypotension)
■ Therapy is largely supportive.
■ Supportive therapy for acute spinal injury
➤ Cardiovascular, respiratory: see above
➤ Immobilize spinal column to prevent further mechanical damage to spinal cord.

> Prevent the development of secondary spinal cord injuries (hypoxemia, hypotension).
- Specific therapy for acute spinal injury
  > Methylprednisolone load (30 mg/kg) IV, then infusion (5.4 mg/kg/hr for 23 hrs)
  > Associated w/ some sensory & motor improvement
  > Other specific therapies not proven (naloxone, TRH, hypothermia, hyperbaric oxygen, catecholamine antagonists, diuretics, calcium channel blockers)
  > Surgery is occasionally needed to achieve alignment, decompress injured spinal cord & stabilize the spine.
- Chronic spinal injury
  > Autonomic: urinary & fecal retention, risk of autonomic hyperreflexia, gastroparesis, poikilothermia
  > Sensory: pts frequently have patchy return of sensation; common to have chronic pain syndrome
  > Motor: depends on level of injury, presence of contractures
  > Psychological: chronic pain syndrome & depression common
- Autonomic hyperreflexia
  > Can develop when spinal shock has resolved & w/ return of spinal cord reflexes
  > Acute generalized autonomic hyperactivity in response to cutaneous or visceral stimuli BELOW spinal cord lesion
  > Stimuli may include distention of bladder, bowel, or intestine; skin stimulation; pyelonephritis; muscle spasm; uterine contractions; surgery.
  > Unlikely if injury is below T10
  > 65–85% of pts w/ level above T7 have autonomic hyperreflexia.
  > Related to lack of supraspinal inhibition on thoracolumbar sympathetic outflow

➤ Stimulus elicits reflex sympathetic activity (if neuro-logically intact, the higher centers would modulate w/ inhibitory impulses).

➤ Sympathetic overactivity BELOW the lesion (hypertension)

➤ Parasympathetic activity ABOVE the lesion (bradycardia, nasal stuffiness, headache, blurred vision, cutaneous vasodilatation)

➤ Mgt: ganglion blocking drugs, alpha blockers (phentolamine), direct-acting vasodilators (nitroprusside), or general or regional anesthesia

STROKE

GEBHARD WAGENER, MD

OVERVIEW

Perioperative stroke

■ Definition

➤ Stroke: cerebral infarction, w/ symptoms lasting >24 hrs

➤ Transient ischemic attack (TIA): symptoms <24 hrs

➤ Reversible ischemic neurologic deficit (RIND): symptoms 24–72 hrs

■ Incidence: 0.02–0.7%

■ Pathophysiology

➤ Mostly thrombotic or embolic

➤ Hypercoagulable state after surgery:

➤ Increase in fibrinogen/factor VII, decrease in AT III

➤ Extended postop bedrest

➤ Dehydration

■ Embolic or thrombotic event leads to decrease in regional cerebral blood flow (CBF) below ischemic threshold (approx. 10 mL/10 g brain tissue/min):

- ➤ Depolarization of membranes & calcium influx
- ➤ Proteolysis
- ➤ Release of excitatory amino acids (glutamate, others)
- ■ Early (intracellular/cytotoxic) & late (extracellular/breakdown of blood-brain barrier) edema leads to ischemic area around focus of stroke (ischemic penumbra/brain at risk).
- ■ Average occurrence: 7 days postop (rarely intraop)
- ■ Increased risk w/:
  - ➤ Age
  - ➤ Previous stroke (1.5–3%)
  - ➤ Kind of surgery
    - • Cardiac surgery (3–5%) > vascular surgery (0.8-3%) > general
  - ➤ Comorbidities
    - • (Asymptomatic) carotid stenosis
    - • Valvular heart disease
    - • Atrial fibrillation
    - • Patent foramen ovale
    - • Hypercoagulability: polycythemia, thrombocytosis, pregnancy, oral contraceptives
    - • Hypertension
    - • Diabetes mellitus
    - • Smoking
    - • Obesity
    - • Prolonged bedrest
- ■ Outcome:
  - ➤ 30% mortality when perioperative
  - ➤ 30% long-term disability
- ■ Musculoskeletal:
  - ➤ Pts w/ stroke:
    - • Evaluate & document deficit prior to surgery.
  - ➤ To prevent perioperative stroke:
    - • Avoid unnecessary bedrest.

FLUIDS AND ELECTROLYTES
- Pts w/ stroke:
  - Malnutrition & dehydration possible: hypernatremia, hyperkalemia
- To prevent perioperative stroke:
  - In pts w/ high risk for perioperative stroke:
    • Ensure adequate hydration: avoid polycythemia

CARDIOPULMONARY
- Pts w/ stroke:
  - Previous stroke risk factor for coronary artery disease
  - Depending on other risk factors, extent of surgery & exercise tolerance: will likely require preop evaluation of myocardial ischemia.
  - Assess baseline BP.
- To prevent perioperative stroke:
  - In pts w/ carotid stenosis:
    • Assess extent of stenosis & baseline BP.
    • Avoid hypotension.

HEMATOLOGIC
- Dehydration can lead to polycythemia & increased blood viscosity.
- Consider aspirin for thrombocytosis.

METABOLIC/NUTRITIONAL
N/A

GASTROINTESTINAL
N/A

NEUROPSYCHIATRIC
- Pts w/ stroke:
  - Pts require early rehab & social & emotional support.
  - Attempt to listen to & understand pts w/ aphasia.

SUBACUTE BACTERIAL ENDOCARDITIS PROPHYLAXIS

JONATHAN T. KETZLER, MD

OVERVIEW
- Etiology
  - Most pts w/ endocarditis have no known predisposing cardiac lesion.
    - There has been a shift from endocarditis predominantly in those w/ rheumatic heart disease, to those w/ congenital heart disease, to those w/ degenerative disease (including mitral valve prolapse) & to those w/ previously normal valves.
  - Pts at risk
    - Structural congenital heart defects
    - Acquired valvular heart disease
    - Endocardial pacemakers
    - Prosthetic valves, conduits, shunts
    - Previous endocarditis
  - Pts not at risk
    - "Innocent" murmurs
    - Nonstructural heart disease (eg, arrhythmias)
  - More likely in pts who use IV drugs & those w/ indwelling catheters or who have undergone cardiac surgery
  - In subacute endocarditis caused by organisms of low virulence, at most 20% follow identifiable medical procedures that cause bacteremias.

FLUID/ELECTROLYTES
N/A

CARDIOPULMONARY
N/A

HEMATOLOGIC
N/A

METABOLIC/NUTRITIONAL
N/A

GASTROINTESTINAL
N/A

NEUROPSYCHIATRIC
N/A

SYSTEMIC LUPUS ERYTHEMATOSUS

ARTHUR ATCHABAHIAN, MD

OVERVIEW
- Autoimmune disease of unclear etiology
  - Genetic factors: association w/ HLA-DR2, -DR3, -A1 & -B8, as well as w/ C2 & C4 complement components deficit
  - More common in black women of childbearing age
  - Most likely related to lymphocyte dysfunction & immune complex formation
- Antibodies against nuclear & cytoplasmic structures are a hallmark of SLE but can be found in other disease.
  - Antibodies to native double-stranded DNA are highly diagnostic for SLE.
- Stresses such as surgery, pregnancy or sepsis can cause exacerbation.
- Drug-induced lupus (essentially caused by procainamide, hydralazine & quinidine), w/ slower progression
- Musculoskeletal
  - Avascular necrosis of femoral head
  - Symmetric arthritis involving hands, wrists, elbows, knees & ankles
  - Proximal myopathy w/ elevated CK

➤ Characteristic malar erythematous rash w/ classically a butterfly shape
  • Present in <50% of pts

FLUIDS AND ELECTROLYTES

■ Glomerulonephritis w/ hematuria & proteinuria, evolving into renal failure
  ➤ Renal involvement in 75% of pts
  ➤ Most commonly diffuse proliferative glomerulonephritis
■ Steroid treatment common

CARDIOPULMONARY

■ Pericarditis common but rarely symptomatic
■ Myocarditis resulting in conduction abnormalities, tachycardia or even CHF
■ Libman-Sacks endocarditis (noninfectious)
  ➤ Involves aortic & mitral valves, usually w/out significant valvular dysfunction
  ➤ Predisposition to bacterial endocarditis & thromboembolic disease
■ Common fetal congenital heart block in children of women w/ lupus
■ Lupus pneumonia
  ➤ Dry cough
  ➤ Dyspnea
  ➤ Fine basilar rales
  ➤ Pleural effusion
  ➤ Diffuse infiltrates on chest x-ray
  ➤ Hypoxemia
  ➤ Restrictive picture on PFTs
  ➤ Possible evolution into acute respiratory failure
  ➤ Difficult to differentiate from infectious pneumonia
  ➤ Diagnosis of elimination
■ Possible progressive pulmonary fibrosis

- High incidence of pulmonary emboli due to hypercoagulable tendency

HEMATOLOGIC
- Autoimmune hemolytic anemia common
  - Warm IgG, occasionally cold IgM
  - Usually responsive to high-dose steroids
  - Other treatment options include immunosuppressive treatment, Danatrol, IVIG or plasmapheresis
- Splenomegaly common; splenectomy sometimes helpful
- Acute immune thrombocytopenia
  - Similar to ITP
  - Initiate IVIG or steroids if platelets <50,000/mm^3
- Rare thrombotic thrombocytopenic purpura
  - Possible hemolytic-uremic syndrome
  - Fever, purpura, microangiopathic hemolytic anemia & renal dysfunction
  - High mortality despite plasmapheresis & high-dose steroids
- Leukopenia common
- Antiphospholipid antibodies
  - Lupus anticoagulant (prolonged PTT but tendency to thrombosis)
  - Anticardiolipin antibody
  - Increased risk of spontaneous abortion
- Increased sensitivity to infection, even w/out steroid or immunosuppressive treatment

METABOLIC-NUTRITIONAL
- Usually normal
- Possible steroid side effects, esp. induced diabetes mellitus

GASTROINTESTINAL
- Abnormal LFTs common

- Lupoid hepatitis w/ recurrent jaundice, hepatomegaly & hyperglobulinemia, possibly fatal
- Possible intestinal ischemia manifesting as acute abdomen
- Possible acute pancreatitis
    - Due to SLE or meds (eg, steroids, azathioprine, thiazide diuretics)
- Possible inflammatory bowel disease w/ ulcerative colitis

NEUROPSYCHIATRIC
- Cerebral "vasculitis" leading to mood disturbances, psychosis, dementia and/or seizures
- Peripheral neuropathy involving cranial & peripheral nerves in 10% of cases
- Rare transverse myelitis w/ paresis or flaccid paralysis of 1 or more limbs
    - Unusual recovery despite early treatment w/ steroids

THALASSEMIA

ARTHUR ATCHABAHIAN, MD

OVERVIEW
- Thalassemia is the result of deletion of one or more genes coding for the alpha (on chromosome 6) or beta (on chromosome 11) subunits of hemoglobin.
- Alpha-thalassemia major (4 deleted alpha genes) is incompatible w/ life & leads to death in utero.
- Hemoglobin H disease (HbH; 3 deleted alpha genes)
    - Limited production of HbF in utero & HbA after birth
    - Hb Bart (4 gamma chains) & Hb H (4 beta chains) precipitate in RBCs, leading to premature destruction in bone marrow & spleen.
- Alpha-thalassemia minor (ATM; 2 deleted alpha genes)

- Alpha-thalassemia 0: Both genes are absent from the same chromosome
- Alpha-thalassemia +: One gene is missing from each chromosome. The + form tends to be slightly more severe, w/ slightly lower hemoglobin levels.
- Alpha-thalassemia silent (1 deleted alpha gene)
  - Minor changes, possible mild anemia
- Beta-thalassemia major (BTM) = Cooley's anemia (both beta genes are deleted)
  - Presence of HbA2 (2 alpha & 2 delta chains) & HbF (2 alpha & 2 gamma chains)
  - Severe anemia develops by 1–2 months, w/ need for chronic transfusion.
  - Need for chelation to prevent hemosiderosis
  - Predominantly in pts of Mediterranean descent
- Beta-thalassemia minor (1 deleted beta gene)
  - Increased production of HbA2 (2 alpha & 2 delta chains)
  - Mild microcytic hypochromic anemia
- Beta-thalassemia major will be discussed in this chapter.

FLUIDS AND ELECTROLYTES
- Usually normal

CARDIOPULMONARY
- CHF possible because of iron overload (less frequent w/ chelation)
- Common SVT & pericarditis
- High sensitivity to digoxin

HEMATOLOGIC
- Microcytic, hypochromic anemia
- Bone marrow hyperactivity
  - Thinning of cortical bone
  - Deformities ("chipmunk face")

- Splenomegaly constant, w/ possible hypersplenism & thrombocytopenia requiring splenectomy

METABOLIC-NUTRITIONAL
- Usually normal

GASTROINTESTINAL
- Liver enlarged because of extramedullary hematopoiesis
  - Possible decreased function & decreased production of coagulation factors

NEUROPSYCHIATRIC
- Spinal cord compression secondary to destruction of vertebral bodies by hyperactive bone marrow is possible.

THYROID AND PARATHYROID DISEASE

GIUDITTA ANGELINI, MD

OVERVIEW
- Thyroid gland
  - Develops from 3rd & 4th branchial arch, descends toward neck
  - Lingual thyroid is in arrested development & potentially only functioning thyroid tissue.
  - Lingual thyroid usually bleeds more profusely w/ biopsy.
- Hypothyroidism
  - Incidence related to amount of iodide in the diet.
  - Incidence: overt 5/1,000, subclinical 15/1,000 in endemic areas
  - Primary hypothyroidism
    - Autoimmune
    - Hashimoto's thyroiditis
    - Irradiation, previous ^{131}I therapy, surgical removal
    - Severe iodine depletion

- Meds: iodines, PTU, methimazole
➤ Secondary hypothyroidism
  - Pituitary
  - Hypothalamic
➤ Symptoms & signs
  - Reduced metabolic activity, cold intolerance, weight gain
  - Lethargy, slow mental function
  - Bradycardia, depressed myocardial contractility, pericardial effusion
  - Delayed tendon reflexes
  - Decreased ventilatory response to hypoxemia/hypercarbia
■ Hyperthyroidism
  ➤ Thyrotoxicosis affects 2% of women, 0.2% of men.
  ➤ Etiology
    - Intrinsic thyroid disease (hyperfunctioning thyroid adenoma, toxic multinodular goiter)
    - Abnormal TSH stimulation (Graves' disease, trophoblastic tumor)
    - Disorders of hormone storage or release (thyroiditis)
    - Excess TSH (pituitary thyrotropin)
    - Extrathyroid (struma ovarii, functioning follicular carcinoma)
    - Exogenous thyroid (iatrogenic, iodine-induced)
  ➤ Most common: multinodular goiter of Graves' disease
  ➤ Symptoms & signs
    - Increased metabolic activity, heat intolerance, night sweats
    - Restlessness, agitation, tremor
    - Palpitations, tachycardia (at rest, sleep), atrial fibrillation
    - Loss of weight

- Goiter
- Parathyroid hormone (PTH)
  - Increases reabsorption of calcium in the kidney; mobilization of calcium from bone
  - Increases renal excretion of phosphate
  - Increases renal clearance & alkalinization of urine
  - Inhibition of renal sodium reabsorption, increased free water clearance
  - Increased vitamin D activity
  - Increased PTH secretion
    - Hypocalcemia & hypomagnesemia
    - Beta-adrenergic agonists
    - Glucocorticoids
- Calcitonin
  - Secreted by parafollicular cells in the thyroid
  - Increases renal excretion of calcium & reabsorption by bone
  - Deficiency in total thyroidectomy & abundance in medullary thyroid cancer
- Primary hyperparathyroidism
  - Incidence
    - About 25/100,000
    - Single adenoma (80%)
    - Multiple adenomata (10–20%)
    - Hyperplasia (9%)
    - Carcinoma (rare)
  - Symptoms & signs
    - Most pts are asymptomatic.
    - Symptoms related to hypercalcemia
      - Polyuria, polydipsia, nephrolithiasis
      - Increased bone resorption
      - Skeletal muscle weakness & fatigability
      - Peptic ulceration & constipation

- Depression, psychosis, confusion, memory loss
- Hypertension, short QTc, heart block, bundle branch block
- Renal manifestations (10%)
- Osteitis fibrosa cystica (rare unless neglected)
- Early surgery decreases morbidity & mortality.

■ Secondary & tertiary hyperparathyroidism
  ➤ Renal disease: impaired hydroxylation of vitamin D leads to:
  ➤ Hypocalcemia, leads to hyperphosphatemia &
  ➤ Parathyroid hyperplasia & autonomous hypersecretion
  ➤ Requires surgical treatment in about 5% of cases in which medical treatment is ineffective

FLUID AND ELECTROLYTES

■ Hypothyroidism
  ➤ Hyponatremia, hypoglycemia
■ Hyperparathyroidism
  ➤ Hypercalcemia: dehydration
  ➤ Nephrolithiasis, nephrocalcinosis
  ➤ Tubular injury
    - Proximal tubular acidosis, aminoaciduria, glycosuria
    - Nephrogenic diabetes insipidus

CARDIOPULMONARY

■ Hypothyroidism
  ➤ Bradycardia, impaired myocardial function
  ➤ Abnormal baroreceptor function
  ➤ Decreased spontaneous ventilation & dyspnea
  ➤ Serous cavity effusions & peripheral edema
  ➤ Angina may be precipitated by rapid thyroid replacement.
■ Hyperthyroidism
  ➤ Palpitations, atrial fibrillation
  ➤ Congestive heart failure, ischemic heart disease
■ Hyperparathyroidism

- Hypertension
- Hypercalcemia: QT prolongation, heart block & bundle branch block

HEMATOLOGIC

- Hypothyroidism
  - Decreased plasma volume
  - Anemia
- Hyperthyroidism
  - Thrombocytopenia

METABOLIC-NUTRITIONAL

- Hypothyroidism
  - Cool, myxedematous extremities
  - Hoarse voice, amenorrhea, hair loss
- Hyperthyroidism
  - Heat intolerance, sweating
  - Gynecomastia
- Hyperparathyroidism
  - Bone loss, but risk of fracture not greatly increased
  - Chondrocalcinosis, pseudogout
  - Juxta-articular erosions, synovitis, periarthritis & pericapsular calcification

GASTROINTESTINAL

- Hypothyroidism
  - Weight gain, poor appetite & constipation
- Hyperthyroidism
  - Weight loss, increased appetite & diarrhea
- Hyperparathyroidism
  - Constipation, peptic ulcer, pancreatitis

NEUROPSYCHIATRIC

- Hypothyroidism
  - Lethargy, weakness, loss of concentration & memory

- ➤ Hearing loss, paresthesias & delayed tendon reflex relaxation
- ➤ Carpal tunnel syndrome
- Hyperthyroidism
  - ➤ Hyperactivity, tremor
  - ➤ Fatigue, weakness, proximal myopathy
- Hyperparathyroidism
  - ➤ Depression, personality changes & memory impairment
  - ➤ Overt psychosis
  - ➤ Obtundation (severe hypercalcemia)

TRANSFUSION THERAPY

DOUGLAS B. COURSIN, MD, AND KARL WILLMANN, MD

OVERVIEW

Roughly 10–12 million units of blood are transfused annually in USA; about 2/3 are administered perioperatively.

- Mainly transfuse blood as component therapy
  - ➤ Packed RBCs
  - ➤ Fresh-frozen plasma (FFP)
  - ➤ Platelets
  - ➤ Cryoprecipitate
  - ➤ Specialized factors
- Use of autologous predonation, acute normovolemic hemodilution w/ reinfusion of the pt's saved blood & cell salvage techniques are alternatives to allogeneic transfusion in selected clinical situations.
  - ➤ Blood substitutes using modified human blood, xenobiotic blood solutions or fluorocarbons are currently investigational.
- Transfusion guidelines as outlined below focus on adults & older children; seek expert advice for premature infants & children <4 months of age. Guidelines continue to evolve.

➤ Major concerns w/ transfusions
- Bloodborne infectious disease
  - Risks continue to decrease but are not zero.
  - HIV, hepatitides, other viral, bacterial, parasitic
- Immune modulation
- Transfusion reaction
- Transfusion-related acute lung injury (TRALI)
- Storage defects

➤ Various organizations have recommendations
- American Society of Anesthesiologists: http://www.asahq.org/publicationsAndServices/blood_component.html
- American Red Cross: http://www.newenglandblood.org/professional/guidelines.htm
- American College of Physicians, American Society of Clinical Pathologists, American Association of Blood Bankers fairly similar

➤ Guidelines must be tailored to the individual pt & his or her clinical circumstances.

➤ Trend is to lower transfusion triggers.

➤ Consider:
- Speed of blood loss/anemia
- Coagulation parameters
- Cardiopulmonary reserve
- If you elect to tolerate a lower Hgb, be certain to ensure adequate volume replacement & intravascular volume.
- Full type & cross-match required to determine compatibility
- Mainly use packed RBCs
  - A unit of packed RBCs will increase the Hgb by 1 g/dL or Hct by about 3% unless the pt is severely anemic, Hct < 20, or actively bleeding.
  - Leukoreduction of RBCs is increasingly performed.

- Usually leukoreduced at the time of donation
- Can do this at the time of administration using special filters, but will slow rate of administration
- Controversial, but many feel leukoreduction limits febrile reactions & may result in improved outcome compared to non-leukoreduced RBCs
- Determine transfusion trigger on an individualized basis.
- Never administer RBCs for volume expansion alone or to enhance wound healing.
- Current guidelines
  - To reverse or treat tissue hypoxia by increasing RBC mass & oxygen delivery
  - Most advocate transfusing normovolemic pts who have Hgb < 7 g/dL.
  - Exceptions
    - Pts w/ active ongoing active blood loss that is unresponsive to crystalloid or colloid infusion
    - Pts w/ acute myocardial ischemia/infarction
    - Pts w/ anemia & CVA
    - Pts w/ symptomatic sickle cell anemia
- ➤ FFP
  - FFP contains all clotting factors.
    - 1 unit of FFP increases clotting factors by about 2.5%.
  - FFP indications
    - Pts w/ documented coagulation factor deficiencies who are actively bleeding or undergoing an invasive procedure w/ significant risk for bleeding
      - Etiologies of coagulopathy
        - Congenital
        - Acquired
          - Liver disease
          - DIC
          - Dilutional

- Anticoagulant use
  - Heparin
  - Warfarin
  - Thrombin inhibitors
- Labs to guide FFP indications
  - INR > 1.5x normal
  - APTT > 1.5x normal
- Management of HUS or TTP
- As part of treatment w/ plasma exchange or plasmapheresis
- Specific plasma protein deficiencies
  - Antithrombin III
  - C-1 esterase
- Platelets
  - Need for platelets may be secondary to quantitative or qualitative defects
    - Thrombocytopenia: low number, quantitative
      - Bone marrow suppression & low production
      - Sequestration (spleen, RES, liver)
      - Destruction
        - Antibody
        - Sepsis
        - Drug-related
    - Thrombocytopathy: abnormal function, qualitative
      - Drug-related
      - Post cardiopulmonary bypass or extracorporeal support
  - Store platelets at room temperature, as opposed to RBCs & FFP.
  - Each unit of platelets contains 60 mL plasma.
  - Platelets may be random donor, single donor or HLA-typed donor.
    - Use depends on indication, availability, underlying pathology & prior exposure to platelets.

- Indications
  - Prevent & treat surgical bleeding
    - Usually aim to transfuse if platelet count < 50,000
    - Some use a threshold of >70–100,000 in pts undergoing ophthalmologic or neurosurgical procedures.
  - High suspicion or lab documentation of qualitative defect
    - Selected bypass pts
    - Selected renal failure pts
    - Reverse effects of drug-induced thrombocytopenia
      - NSAIDs
      - ASA
      - Antiplatelet drugs
        - Persantine
        - Glycoprotein IIb/IIIA inhibitors
        - Other
  - Platelets should not be transfused in pts w/ heparin-induced thrombocytopenia (HIT), idiopathic thrombocytopenia (ITP), TTP, HUS, or post-transfusion purpura unless there is life-threatening bleeding (suggest hematology guidance).
- Cryoprecipitate
  - Indications
    - Consult hematology for mgt of coagulation disorders such as hemophilia, vWf deficiency & other rare coagulopathies or hypercoagulable state.
    - Fibrinogen < 100 mg/dL
    - Factor VIII, IX or vWf deficiency
    - As part of fibrin glue local application
- Special products
  - CMV-negative products (use only if the recipient is CMV-negative)
    - Stem cell or solid organ transplant pt
    - Pregnant woman

- AIDS, severe immunosuppression, Hodgkin's
- Status post splenectomy
- Irradiated cells
  - Stem cell recipient
  - Intrauterine transfusions
  - Directed donation blood from a relative
  - Severe immunosuppression, AIDS, Hodgkin's, pt undergoing high-dose chemotherapy or radiation therapy
  - Recipients of HLA-matched platelets
- Factor VIIa
  - Currently available for patients w/ factor VII deficiency
  - Some case reports of broader use in the bleeding pt
- Special considerations
  - Suspected transfusion reaction
    - May be acute or delayed
    - If you suspect an immediate reaction:
      - Stop the transfusion.
      - Symptoms may range from minor, such as fever, to shock, hematuria, DIC, etc.
      - Supportive care directed at specific type of reaction suspected
      - Clerical check
      - Send both anticoagulated & clotted blood samples from pt to lab for evaluation, along w/ suspected blood product.
      - Send urinalysis to lab.
      - Communicate w/ blood bank about results & need for additional information or testing.
      - No further transfusion of blood products unless life-threatening hemorrhage & until cleared by blood bank
  - Transfusion-related acute lung injury (TRALI)
    - http://www.fda.gov/cber/ltr/trali101901.htm

- http://www.google.com/search?hl=en&ie=ISO-8859-1&q=TRALI
  - See [PDF] Transfusion Related Acute Lung Injury (TRALI)
- Relatively rare (0.02% of all transfusions), but a major cause of post-transfusion morbidity & mortality
- Results in part from an antibody response of the donor to recipient WBCs
- Donor most often multiparous woman
  - Often, not always, HLA sensitized
- May require "second hit" from hypoxia or other not fully understood recipient factors
- Develops within 1–6 hrs of transfusion, may be as late as 24 hrs
- All blood products may cause
- Rapid onset of acute respiratory insufficiency
  - Dyspnea, shortness of breath, cyanosis, hypotension, fever & pulmonary edema may develop.
  - No definitive test to establish diagnosis; one of exclusion
  - Chest x-ray often shows diffuse infiltrates.
  - Rule out cardiogenic or volume overload.
  - Treatment is supportive.
    - Stop current blood transfusion if suspected.
    - Oxygen, noninvasive or invasive ventilatory support
  - Report it to your blood bank.

FLUID AND ELECTROLYTES

▪ Transfuse through normal saline-containing infusions to avoid hemolysis, crenation or chelation of anticoagulant.

CARDIOPULMONARY

▪ Transfusion trigger for pts w/ acute coronary syndrome or acute MI is Hgb 10–11.

HEMATOLOGIC

N/A

METABOLIC-NUTRITIONAL

N/A

GASTROINTESTINAL

- Renal compromise is a complication of transfusion reaction from pigment; diuresis & supportive care are needed.

NEUROPSYCHIATRIC

N/A

VON WILLEBRAND'S DISEASE

KARL WILLMANN, MD, AND D. B. COURSIN, MD

OVERVIEW

- von Willebrand's disease is a bleeding diathesis character-ized by mucocutaneous bleeding, epistaxis, menorrhagia, easy bruising & prolonged bleeding time. It is an autosomal dominant genetic disease representing a deficiency or defect of von Willebrand factor (vWf).
- Clear family history not always present, as disease severity varies substantially
- vWf has several roles in the coagulation cascade, including protecting factor VIII from degradation & binding of platelets to damaged endothelium.
- Platelet numbers are normal & PTT is normal unless severe disease. PT is normal.
- Of the inherited bleeding disorders, it is the most common.
- There are 5 subtypes of von Willebrand's disease.
- The diagnosis is made by antigen immunoassay of vWf:Ag & ristocetin cofactor activity (vWf:Co). Along w/ immunoassays, immunoelectrophoresis distinguishes between the different

types. There are several multimers of different sizes that make up vWf.

> Type I: Most common. Decreased vWf:Ag & vWf:Co; normal multimers, just decreased number.

> Type IIa: Decreased vWf:Ag & greatly decreased vWf:Co w/ decrease in medium & large multimers

> Type IIb: Decreased vWf:Ag & near-normal vWf:Co; abnormal large multimers that bind to platelets w/out normal activity

> Type III: No vWf:Ag or vWf:Co, no vWf present

> Type IV: Decreased vWf:Ag & vWf:Co, w/ normal vWf, but platelet GPIb receptor binds only large multimers

FLUID AND ELECTROLYTES
- No special concerns

CARDIOPULMONARY
- No special concerns

HEMATOLOGIC
- There are several types; see "Overview." Pt may have had previous transfusions of coagulation factors for excessive bleeding. These pts are at risk for virally transmitted diseases such as hepatitis & HIV.

METABOLIC-NUTRITIONAL
- No special concerns

GASTROINTESTINAL
- Pts who have received factor therapy from random donors are at risk for hepatitis & its sequelae.

NEUROPSYCHIATRIC
- No special concerns

PART TWO

Pharmacology

ADRENAL & PITUITARY DISEASE

GIUDITTA ANGELINI, MD

PHARMACOLOGY

- Bromocriptine
  - Dopamine agonist
  - First-line treatment for prolactinoma
  - Potential treatment for acromegaly (primary treatment surgical): start at 1 mg qd & titrate against prolactin concentration to 5–15 mg qd.
  - Alternative therapy: cabergoline
  - Monitor visual field defects during therapy.
  - Medical therapy curative in 95% of cases, w/ regression of visual field defects in 75% of cases
  - No evidence of teratogenicity, but usually stopped during pregnancy
  - Surgery indicated after failure or intolerance to medical therapy
- Somatostatin
  - Potential treatment for acromegaly (see bromocriptine)
- Metyrapone, betaconazole
  - Reverse side effects of increased concentrations of circulating cortisol
- Surgery is primary therapy in:
  - Acromegaly
  - ACTH tumors
  - TSH adenomas
  - Gonadotroph adenomas

DRUG DOSING
N/A

ADULT CONGENITAL HEART DISEASE

MARY E. McSWEENEY, MD

PHARMACOLOGY

■ Negative inotropic & chronotropic agents
  ➤ Use to decrease outflow obstruction in pts w/ subvalvular stenosis.
  ➤ Avoid in pts w/ high PVR: result in increased R-to-L shunt
■ Vasodilators
  ➤ Avoid in pts w/ high PVR: result in increased R-to-L shunt
■ Alpha-adrenergic agonists
  ➤ Use in pts w/ shunts & high PVR to maintain diastolic perfusion pressure, increase SVR & prevent increased R-to-L shunt.

DRUG DOSING
N/A

ALCOHOL ABUSE

JONATHAN T. KETZLER, MD

PHARMACOLOGY

■ Mechanisms of alcohol-induced CNS depression
  ➤ Potentiates gamma-aminobutyric acid (GABA) (inhibitory amino acid)
  ➤ Inhibits n-methyl-D-aspartate (NMDA) (excitatory amino acid)
■ Also acts on noradrenergic, dopaminergic, serotoninergic & opioid pathways
■ Chronic exposure: decreased GABA synthesis, increased NMDA synthesis

- Abrupt withdrawal: relative lack of GABA, relative excess of NMDA
- Alcohol withdrawal may cause kindling:
  - Repeated exposures to electric/chemical stimuli cause progressively exaggerated neuronal response (kindling).
  - Repeated withdrawal over time leads to increased CNS excitability (exacerbated withdrawal syndrome).
    - Anti-kindling agents such as carbamazepine (Tegretol) are effective in treating alcohol withdrawal syndrome, esp. anxiety & agitation.

DRUG DOSING
- N/A

ANEMIA

DOUGLAS B. COURSIN, MD AND KARL WILLMANN, MD

PHARMACOLOGY
- Little effect on pharmacology other than changes w/ associated abnormal binding proteins & end-organ pathology in liver or kidney
- Hemolysis may damage kidneys.

DRUG DOSING
- Little effect on drug dosing unless associated abnormal binding proteins or end-organ pathology in liver or kidney

---

ANKYLOSING SPONDYLITIS

HUGH R. PLAYFORD, MD

PHARMACOLOGY
N/A

DRUG DOSING
N/A

ANTICOAGULATION THERAPY

JONATHAN T. KETZLER, MD

PHARMACOLOGY
N/A

DRUG DOSING
N/A

AORTIC REGURGITATION

ROBERT N. SLADEN, MD

PHARMACOLOGY
- Chronotropic, inotropic agents are useful.
  - Tachycardia helps maintain forward CO (shorter diastolic regurgitant time).
  - Increased contractility compensates for regurgitant fraction.
- Avoid negative inotropic & chronotropic agents:
  - Decrease cardiac output
  - Slower heart rate increases diastolic regurgitant time.
- Avoid alpha-adrenergic agents:
  - Increase SVR & regurgitation
- Vasodilator agents may decrease SVR & increase forward ejection:
  - Limited by decreased diastolic in perfusion pressure, impaired MVO_2
- Common maintenance meds & side effects
  - Digoxin (digitoxic conduction disorders, arrhythmias)

➤ Loop diuretics (hypokalemia, hyponatremia)
➤ Coumadin (bleeding)

DRUG DOSING
N/A

AORTIC STENOSIS

ROBERT N. SLADEN, MD

PHARMACOLOGY

■ Negative inotropic & chronotropic agents can decrease gradient, improve MVO_2
    ➤ Beta blockers (metoprolol, esmolol)
    ➤ Calcium channel blockers (verapamil, diltiazem)
■ Alpha-adrenergic agents can support diastolic perfusion pressure during hypotension
    ➤ Phenylephrine (pure alpha-agonist) increases SVR, reflex bradycardia (preferred).
    ➤ Norepinephrine (mixed agent) increases contractility (avoid).
■ Avoid chronotropic, inotropic agents
    ➤ Increased contractility increases pressure gradient across aortic valve
    ➤ Tachycardia decreases diastolic fill time, impairs MVO_2
    ➤ May precipitate angina, syncope, sudden death
■ Avoid vasodilator agents
    ➤ Decrease diastolic perfusion pressure, impair MVO_2
    ➤ Increase gradient across aortic valve
    ➤ Adverse effects exacerbated by reflex tachycardia
■ Use diuretics w/ care (excess decreases preload)
■ Common maintenance meds & side effects
    ➤ Beta blockers (bronchoconstriction)
    ➤ Calcium channel blockers (low cardiac output)

DRUG DOSING
N/A

BRONCHOSPASTIC DISEASE

HUGH PLAYFORD, MD

PHARMACOLOGY
- Usually unchanged
- No evidence of tolerance to beta-2 agonists w/ chronic treatment

DRUG DOSING
N/A

CARCINOID SYNDROME

GIUDITTA ANGELINI, MD

PHARMACOLOGY
- Octreotide
- Steroids
  - Treat bronchospasm
- Theophyllines
  - Treat bronchospasm
- Aprotinin
  - Treat flushing & hypotension
- Ondansetron
- Ranitidine/Benadryl

DRUG DOSING
- Octreotide
  - Half-life 160 min
  - 50–500 mcg SQ q8h can be administered as maintenance

➤ 10–300 mcg/hr IV continuous infusion

➤ When discontinued, weaning must occur over 1 wk.

CHEMOTHERAPEUTIC AGENTS

JONATHAN T. KETZLER, MD

SCREENING AND EVALUATION

■ Anthracyclines

➤ There are no tests to determine which pts will develop heart failure.

➤ Do gated radionucleotide blood pooled study or echocardiogram as baseline before patient receives a cumulative dose of 400 mg/m^2 & before each following treatment.

➤ Because injury can continue for years after treatment, ideally a full cardiac evaluation should be done within 1 month of elective surgery.

■ Bleomycin

➤ Chest x-ray & pulmonary function tests to evaluate for pneumonitis & pulmonary fibrosis

DRUG DOSING

N/A

CHRONIC OBSTRUCTIVE PULMONARY DISEASE (COPD)

HUGH R. PLAYFORD, MBBS

PHARMACOLOGY

Minimal change

DRUG DOSING

N/A

CHRONIC RENAL FAILURE

ROBERT N. SLADEN, MD

PHARMACOLOGY
- Most IV anesthetic agents are lipid-soluble & non-ionized
  - Hepatic biotransformation to active or inactive water-soluble metabolites
  - Excreted in bile or urine
- Lipid-insoluble, highly ionized drugs (mostly muscle relaxants)
  - Directly excreted by kidney
- Renal disease alters anesthetic & parenteral drug clearance:
  - Decreased blood flow (drug delivery)
  - Increased unbound free fraction of highly protein-bound drugs (hypoalbuminemia, acidosis)
  - Decreased enzymes & transport processes that remove drug from blood
- Duration of action (bolus or short-lived infusion)
  - Dependent on redistribution, not elimination
  - Loading dose is not decreased (unless unbound free fraction increased).
  - Maintenance doses decreased (drug accumulates w/ repeated dosing)
- Pharmacodynamics altered even if pharmacokinetics not changed
  - Pts are debilitated, w/ depleted lean body mass.
  - Risk of respiratory depression (opioid or volatile anesthetics)
- Reduce all drug dosages by 25–50%.

DRUG DOSING
- Drugs independent of renal function for elimination
  - Enzymatic or spontaneous breakdown in the blood
  - Accumulation is unlikely

- Examples
  - Succinylcholine
  - Atracurium, cisatracurium
  - Remifentanil
  - Esmolol
- Drugs w/ increased unbound fraction in hypoalbuminemia
  - Increased free or active fraction
  - Decrease doses 20–50% (depends on severity of hypoalbuminemia)
- Examples
  - Thiopental
  - Methohexital
  - Diazepam
- Drugs predominantly dependent on renal elimination
  - Loading doses remain unaltered
  - Eliminate or decrease maintenance dose.
- Examples
  - Gallamine, metubine
  - Digoxin
  - Penicillins, cephalosporins, aminoglycosides, vancomycin
  - Cyclosporine A
- Drugs partially dependent on renal elimination
  - Decrease maintenance doses by 30–50%.
  - Titrate carefully to effect.
- Examples
  - Anticholinergic, cholinergic agents
  - Pancuronium, pipecuronium
  - Vecuronium, rocuronium, doxacurium
  - Milrinone, amrinone
  - Phenobarbital
  - Aprotinin, aminocaproic acid, tranexamic acid
- Drugs w/ active metabolites that are renally eliminated
  - Prolonged effect despite rapid hepatic biotransformation of parent compound

➤ Decrease maintenance doses by 30–50%, or avoid altogether.
- Examples
  ➤ Morphine (morphine-3-glucuronide, morphine-6-glucuronide, normorphine)
  ➤ Meperidine (normeperidine)
  ➤ Diazepam (desmethyldiazepam, oxazepam)
  ➤ Midazolam (l-hydroxymidazolam)
  ➤ Pancuronium (3-hydroxypancuronium)
  ➤ Vecuronium (desacetylvecuronium)
  ➤ Sevoflurane, enflurane (fluoride)
  ➤ Sodium nitroprusside (thiocyanate)

COCAINE TOXICITY

MARY E. McSWEENEY, MD

PHARMACOLOGY

- Benzoylmethylecgonine (cocaine)
  ➤ Crystalline form: made by dissolving alkaloid in hydrochloric acid; forms water-soluble salt (usual street cocaine)
  ➤ Crack: unpurified freebase cocaine: formed by combining cocaine hydrochloride w/ sodium bicarbonate & cooking in water; makes an oil-like substance that separates from water & forms small pieces (rocks), which can be smoked
  ➤ Freebase: ether extracted (rarely used)
- Absorption: absorbed from mucus membranes & respiratory, GI & GU tracts
- Onset: peak effect inhaled (smoked) 1–3 minutes, IV route 3–5 minutes, intranasal route 20 minutes, GI route up to 90 minutes
- Half-life: IV or inhalational administration associated w/ a 60-minute half-life, vasoconstriction associated w/ the intranasal route prolongs the half-life to 2–3 hrs

■ Metabolism: by plasma & hepatic cholinesterase & nonenzymatic hydrolysis to inactive water-soluble metabolites (benzoylecgonine, ecgonine methyl ester), which are excreted in the urine along with a small amount (10–20%) of unchanged cocaine. Those w/ decreased cholinesterase activity (fetuses, infants, pregnant women, elderly, patients w/ liver disease or pseudocholinesterase deficiency) are at higher risk.

DRUG DOSING
N/A

CONGESTIVE HEART FAILURE

MUHAMMED ITANI, MD, AND JONATHAN T. KETZLER, MD

PHARMACOLOGY
■ Angiotensin-converting enzyme inhibitors (ACEI)
  ➤ Drugs
    • Captopril (short acting)
    • Enalapril(at) (intermediate acting, only IV ACEI)
    • Lisinopril, ramipril (long acting)
  ➤ Alleviate symptoms & prolong survival
  ➤ Affect remodeling of the myocardium
  ➤ Relieve symptoms & conserve potassium
■ Diuretics
  ➤ Drugs
    • Medullary thick ascending loop (mTAL): furosemide, bumetanide, torsemide, ethacrynic acid
    • Distal tubule: hydrochlorothiazide, metolazone
    • Distal tubule, collecting duct (potassium-sparing): aldosterone antagonists: spironolactone
  ➤ Relieve circulatory & pulmonary congestion
  ➤ Decrease atrial & ventricular diastolic pressures & wall stress; improve subendocardial perfusion

- ➤ K^+ supplementation may be needed (loop, thiazide diuretics).
- ➤ Hyperkalemia may occur w/ K-sparing diuretics (spironolactone).
- ➤ Hypovolemia, prerenal azotemia & low cardiac output may occur.
- ■ Oral vasodilators
  - ➤ Prazosin (alpha-antagonist)
- ■ IV vasodilators
  - ➤ Arterial dilators (afterload reduction): dihydropyridine calcium blockers (nicardipine)
  - ➤ Venodilators (preload reduction): NTG
  - ➤ Balanced vasodilators (arterial + venous dilation): SNP, nesiritide
  - ➤ Relax both arterial & venous vessels & improve stroke volume & decrease LV pressure; useful in diastolic dysfunction
- ■ Digoxin
  - ➤ Actions
    - • Enhances inotropy & decreases activation of sympathetic nervous system
    - • Dose by level in CHF w/ SR (0.5–1.5 ng/mL): dose-dependent inotropy
    - • Dose by ventricular rate in AF; seek subtoxic AV block
    - • Decrease maintenance dose in renal insufficiency
  - ➤ Toxicity
    - • Exacerbated by hypokalemia, hypercalcemia, hypomagnesemia
    - • Symptoms: anorexia, nausea
    - • Dysrhythmias (sinus bradycardia, PAT w/ block, V bigeminy, refractory VT)
    - • Treat w/ correction of predisposing factor: atropine (bradycardia); lidocaine, phenytoin (VT).

➤ Anesthetic planning w/ digoxin toxicity
  • Delay elective surgery.
  • Consider digoxin antibodies.
  • Avoid sympathomimetic drugs (ketamine) & calcium.
  • Avoid high levels of volatile agents.
  • Avoid hyperventilation (ie, respiratory alkalosis & hypokalemia).
  • Administer K for tachyarrhythmias (w/ normal renal function & absence of heart block)
  • SB: atropine; VT: lidocaine, phenytoin (may be refractory to cardioversion)

DRUG DOSING
N/A

COR PULMONALE AND RHF

MUHAMMED ITANI, MD, AND JONATHAN T. KETZLER, MD

PHARMACOLOGY
■ Volatile anesthetic agents
  ➤ Well-tolerated, potent bronchodilators
■ N_2O
  ➤ AVOID: induces pulmonary vasoconstriction, may worsen pulmonary hypertension
■ Inhaled nitric oxide
  ➤ Specific pulmonary vasodilator
  ➤ May help decrease pulmonary arterial pressure
■ Neuromuscular blocking agents (NMBA)
  ➤ May be used safely in pts w/ RV failure
■ Intravenous induction agents (propofol, thiopental)
  ➤ AVOID or use slowly & cautiously.
  ➤ May induce severe systemic hypotension (uncompensated w/ fixed pulmonary vasoconstriction)

- Opioids & sedatives
  - ➤ Use extreme caution, esp. preoperatively & in awake pts.
  - ➤ Risk of hypoventilation & worsening of arterial hypoxemia

DRUG DOSING
- Altered, depending on severity of hepatic or renal failure

DIABETES MELLITUS AND DIABETIC EMERGENCIES

DOUGLAS B. COURSIN, MD

PHARMACOLOGY
- Most routine meds can be given prior to surgery; in particular, beta blockers, meds to decrease gastric acid (H2 blockers, proton pump inhibitors). ACE inhibitors are usually held the day of surgery to avoid hypotension.
- Hold oral hypoglycemic agents the day of surgery, although acarbose can be administered.
- Insulin
  - ➤ Type 1 diabetics always require some basal insulin.
  - ➤ Obtain a fasting blood sugar prior to administering preop insulins.
  - ➤ Regular is routinely held, unless blood glucose > 250 mg/dL.
- Any pharmacokinetic changes usually secondary to advanced renal disease

DRUG DOSING
- Insulin
  - ➤ Ultra-short, short, intermediate, long acting
  - ➤ Vary as to onset of action & duration
  - ➤ Often given as split doses
    - AM & PM
    - Given as boluses of ultra-short or short-acting agents w/ meals

- ➤ For perioperative use
  - Regular is usually held
  - 1/2 to 2/3 of the normal intermediate-acting agents are given on the day of surgery w/ appropriate IV access & glucose monitoring & supplementation
  - Glargine is peakless, given in the PM, can be given the night before surgery & then additional supplementation
- ➤ Ultrashort acting
  - Lispro or aspart, not used intraoperatively
- ➤ Short acting
  - Regular: preparation used for continuous insulin infusion
  - Otherwise usually hold day of surgery to avoid hypoglycemia
- ➤ Intermediate to long acting
  - NPH
  - Lente
- ➤ Long acting
  - Ultralente
  - Glargine
- ■ Administered at nighttime
- ■ Peakless
- ■ Oral hypoglycemic agents: hold day of surgery
  - ➤ Do not restart metformin postop until sure that renal & hepatic functions are adequate.

EPILEPSY

GEBHARD WAGENER, MD

PHARMACOLOGY

- ■ Liver enzyme induction (cytochrome P450) by carbamazepine, phenytoin, barbiturates

- Increased resistance to neuromuscular blocking agents (esp. phenytoin)
- Carbamazepine & phenytoin levels may be elevated up to 1 wk postop.
- Except for gabapentin: hepatic elimination

DRUG DOSING
N/A

THE GERIATRIC PATIENT

HUGH R. PLAYFORD, MD

PHARMACOLOGY

Pharmacokinetics
- Usually manifest as increased elimination half-life
  - Decreased renal clearance (digoxin, antibiotics, pancuronium)
  - Increased hepatic clearance (propranolol, lidocaine, vecuronium)
  - Increased volume of distribution (diazepam) related to increased total fat content & decreased serum albumin
  - Leads to accumulation of drugs (and /or metabolites) & increased incidence of adverse events

Pharmacodynamics
- In general, decreased responsiveness of receptors (esp. catecholamines)
- Neuromuscular junction receptors unchanged w/ aging

Elimination
- Renal dysfunction will prolong the elimination half-lives of renally metabolized & eliminated drugs.
- Hepatic dysfunction will prolong the elimination half-lives of hepatically metabolized & eliminated drugs.

DRUG DOSING
N/A

GI DISEASE

GEBHARD WAGENER, MD

PHARMACOLOGY
- Oral bioavailability erratic w/ GI disease
- Protein loss common w/ enteropathies
- Dehydration causes decreased blood volume.

DRUG DOSING
N/A

HEMOGLOBINOPATHIES

DOUGLAS B. COURSIN, MD, AND KARL WILLMANN, MD

PHARMACOLOGY
- Little effect on pharmacology other than changes w/ associated abnormal binding proteins & end-organ pathology in liver or kidney
- Hemolysis may damage kidneys.

DRUG DOSING
- Little effect on drug dosing unless associated abnormal binding proteins or end-organ pathology in liver or kidney

---

HEMOPHILIA A & HEMOPHILIA B

KARL WILLMANN, MD, AND D. B. COURSIN, MD

PHARMACOLOGY
- No special concerns

DRUG DOSING

- Pts w/ hepatitis & liver dysfunction require drug dosing appropriate to the degree of liver failure.

HERBAL THERAPY

JONATHAN T. KETZLER, MD

PHARMACOLOGY

- **Cayenne (*Capsicum annuum*)**
  - Other names: cayenne, chili pepper, paprika
  - Uses
    - External: muscle soreness
    - Internal: GI distress
  - Issues
    - May cause blisters when applied topically
    - May cause hypothermia when used internally
- **Danshen (*Salvia miltiorrhiza*)**
  - Other names: tanshen, red sage, red ginseng, Chinese sage
  - Uses
    - Ischemic heart disease
    - Atherosclerotic disease
    - Antioxidant
    - Antihypertensive
  - Issues
    - May cause bleeding
- **Dong quai (*Angelica sinensis*)**
  - Other names: dang gui, tang kuei
  - Uses
    - The "ultimate herb" for women
    - Restores menstrual regularity & hormonal balance
    - Blood thinner
    - Antiarrhythmic

- Hematopoietic
- Antioxidant
➤ Issues
  - May cause bleeding

■ **Echinacea (*Echinacea purpurea*)**
➤ Other names: purple cone flower
➤ Uses
  - Colds, urinary tract infections, bronchitis, topically for wounds & burns
➤ Issues
  - May cause inflammation of liver if used w/ certain other meds, such as anabolic steroids or methotrexate
  - May decrease the effectiveness of corticosteroids

■ **Ephedra (*Ephedra sinica*)**
➤ Other names: ephedrine, ma-huang, Chinese joint fir
➤ Uses
  - Over-the-counter diet pills
  - Added energy
  - Bacteriostatic
  - Antitussive
➤ Issues
  - In late December 2003, FDA banned ephedra from the marketplace because of health concerns.
  - Arrhythmias
  - May interact w/ certain antidepressants or certain BP meds to cause dangerous elevations in BP or heart rate
  - Enhanced sympathomimetic effects when used w/ MAO inhibitors
  - Hypertension when used w/ oxytocin
  - May cause stroke or death in certain individuals

■ **Feverfew (*Tanacetum parthenium*)**
➤ Other names: featherfew, midsummer daisy
➤ Uses
  - Migraines
  - Antipyretic

- Anxiety
- Joint stiffness
➤ Issues
  - Platelet inhibition
  - Rebound headache
  - 5–15% of users develop aphthous ulcers & GI upset.
■ **Garlic (*Allium sativum*)**
➤ Other names: clove garlic, ajo
➤ Uses
  - Lower lipids
  - Lower BP
  - Antiplatelet
  - Antioxidant
  - Blood thinner
➤ Issues
  - Enhances effect of warfarin
  - May decrease effectiveness of AIDS therapy, especially saquinavir
■ **Ginger (*Zingiber officinale*)**
➤ Other names: black ginger, African ginger
➤ Uses
  - Antiemetic
  - Antispasmodic
➤ Issues
  - May increase bleeding by inhibiting thromboxane synthetase
  - Increased sedation
■ **Ginkgo (*Gingko biloba*)**
➤ Other names: maidenhair tree, fossil tree
➤ Uses: circulatory stimulant
➤ Issues: may increase bleeding, especially in pts already taking certain anti-clotting meds
■ **Ginseng (*Panax ginseng*)**
➤ Other names: American ginseng, Chinese ginseng, Korean ginseng

- Uses
  - Energy enhancer
  - Aphrodisiac
  - Antioxidant
- Issues
  - Decreased effectiveness of warfarin
  - Somnolence
  - Hypertonia
  - Edema
  - Tachycardia
  - Enhanced response to sympathomimetics
  - Postmenopausal bleeding
  - Mania in pts on phenelzine
- **Goldenseal (*Hydrastis canadensis*)**
  - Other names: orange root, yellow root, ground raspberry, tumeric root, eye root
  - Uses
    - Diuretic
    - Anti-inflammatory
    - Laxative
    - Hemostatic
  - Issues
    - Overdose may cause paralysis.
    - Causes excretion of free water, not sodium
    - May worsen edema
    - May worsen hypertension
- **Kava-Kava (*Methysticum*)**
  - Other names: kawa awa pepper
  - Uses: anxiolytic
  - Issues
    - May enhance the sedative effects of anesthesia
    - May increase the effects of certain anti-seizure meds
    - May cause serious liver injury
    - May worsen the symptoms of Parkinson's disease

- Can enhance the effects of alcohol
- May increase the risk of suicide in pts w/ certain types of depression

■ **Licorice (*Glycyrrhiza glabra*)**
  ➤ Other names: licorice root, sweet root
  ➤ Uses
    - GI ulcers
    - Antitussive
    - Bronchitis
    - Most licorice candy contains little or no herbal licorice, but check product ingredients ("licorice flavoring" is safer than "licorice extract," or "natural licorice").
  ➤ Issues
    - May increase BP
    - May cause hypokalemia
    - May increase swelling
    - Contraindicated in hepatic & renal insufficiency

■ **Milk Thistle (*Silmarin*)**
  ➤ Uses: liver disease
  ➤ Issues
    - Should be no issues if taken as directed
    - Has caused diarrhea in animals
    - One case of urticaria reported in Russia

■ **Saw Palmetto (*Serenoa repens*)**
  ➤ Other names: sabal, cabbage palm
  ➤ Uses
    - Benign prostatic hypertrophy
    - Anti-androgenic
  ➤ Issues: interferes w/ hormone therapy

■ **St. John's Wort (*Hypericum perforatum*)**
  ➤ Other names: hardhay, amber goatweed
  ➤ Uses
    - Antidepressant
    - Anxiolytic

➤ Issues
- May enhance the sedative effects of anesthesia
- Enhanced sympathomimetic effects when used w/ MAO inhibitors
- May cause photosensitivity

■ **Valerian (*Valeriana officinalis*)**
  ➤ Other names: all heal, setwall, vandal root
  ➤ Uses
  - Sedative
  - Anxiolytic
  ➤ Issues: may enhance the sedative effects of anesthesia

DRUG DOSING
N/A

HIV & AIDS

GEBHARD WAGENER, MD

PHARMACOLOGY

HAART (highly active antiretroviral therapy)
■ Nucleoside reverse transcriptase inhibitors (NRTIs): anemia, neutropenia, induction of liver enzymes
  ➤ AZT, didanosine, lamivudine
■ Non-nucleoside reverse transcriptase inhibitors (NNRTIs): induce cytochrome P450,
  ➤ Nevirapine, efavirenz
■ Protease inhibitors (PIs): inhibit cytochrome P-450, CAD, hyperglycemia, may prolong fentanyl half-life
  ➤ Saquinavir, ritonavir, nelfinavir
■ Benzodiazepines & opioids: increased sensitivity w/ AIDS dementia
■ Neuroleptics: extrapyramidal symptoms more likely

DRUG DOSING
N/A

HYPERTENSION

MUHAMMED ITANI, MD AND JONATHAN T. KETZLER, MD

PHARMACOLOGY
N/A

DRUG DOSING
N/A

ICU PATIENT SCHEDULED FOR INTERCURRENT SURGERY

DOUGLAS B. COURSIN, MD

PHARMACOLOGY
- Altered pharmacokinetics/dynamics
  - Bioavailability via enteric & subcutaneous route unpredictable
  - Both PK & PD can be unpredictable
  - Limited data for some medication use in ICU pts
  - End-organ dysfunction
    - Renal
    - Hepatic
    - Combined renal/hepatic
  - Altered receptor function
  - Drug compatibility
    - Do you have adequate access to infuse all of the drugs & anesthetic agents needed?
  - ICU pts receive an average of 10–15 meds; chance of drug interaction is high.

DRUG DOSING

- Titrate to effect
- Volume of distribution may be significantly altered, especially in renal/hepatic dysfunction, hypoalbuminemic state.
  - ➤ May require larger doses for effect (eg, nondepolarizing agents)
  - ➤ Clearance may be prolonged.
  - ➤ Take into account changes in kinetics of highly protein-bound meds.
- Concurrent pathology may create agonist or antagonistic response to meds.

IDIOPATHIC HYPERTROPHIC SUBAORTIC STENOSIS (IHSS)

ROBERT N. SLADEN, MD

PHARMACOLOGY

- Negative inotropic & chronotropic agents can decrease gradient, improve MVO_2
  - ➤ Beta blockers (metoprolol, esmolol)
  - ➤ Calcium channel blockers (verapamil, diltiazem)
- Alpha-adrenergic agents can support diastolic perfusion pressure during hypotension
  - ➤ Phenylephrine (pure alpha-agonist) increases SVR, reflex bradycardia (preferred).
  - ➤ Norepinephrine (mixed agent) increases contractility (avoid).
- Avoid chronotropic, inotropic agents
  - ➤ Increased contractility increases pressure gradient across aortic valve.
  - ➤ Tachycardia decreases diastolic fill time, impairs MVO_2
  - ➤ May precipitate angina, syncope, sudden death

- Avoid vasodilator agents
  - Decrease diastolic perfusion pressure, impair MVO_2
  - Increase gradient across aortic valve
  - Adverse effects exacerbated by reflex tachycardia
- Use diuretics w/ care (excess decreases preload).
- Common maintenance meds & side effects
  - Beta blockers (bronchoconstriction)
  - Calcium channel blockers (low cardiac output)

DRUG DOSING
N/A

ISCHEMIC HEART DISEASE

MUHAMMED ITANI, MD, AND JONATHAN T. KETZLER, MD

PHARMACOLOGY
- Antiplatelet drugs
  - Drugs
    - Aspirin
    - Clopidogrel (Plavix)
    - Platelet glycoprotein IIb/IIIa receptor inhibitors (abciximab)
  - Indications
    - Decrease risk of cardiac events in pts w/ IHD
    - During AMI w/ pain onset
    - Placement of coronary artery stents
- Nitrates
  - Drugs
    - Nitroglycerine (sublingual, IV, spray, ointment, patch)
    - Isosorbide
  - Advantages
    - May decrease frequency, duration & severity of angina
    - May increase exercise tolerance

- Decrease myocardial preload & afterload
- Decrease myocardial oxygen consumption
- Vasodilate coronaries & collaterals
➤ Limitations
  - Rapid tolerance w/ sustained therapy
  - Hypotension & headaches
■ Beta blockers
  ➤ Drugs
    - Long acting: nadolol (non-selective), atenolol (beta-1 selective), sotalol
    - Intermediate acting: propranolol (non-selective), metoprolol (beta-1 selective)
    - Short acting: esmolol (beta-1 selective)
  ➤ Advantages
    - Decrease myocardial oxygen consumption by decreasing contractility
    - Increase myocardial perfusion by decreasing heart rate & increasing diastolic time
    - Very beneficial for pts w/ stable angina
    - Decrease risk of death & reinfarction in pts w/ history of previous MI
    - Should be given as early as possible in patients w/ AMI
  ➤ Side effects
    - Beta-2 antagonism (bronchospasm, exacerbate peripheral vascular disease)
    - Excessive myocardial depression (worsened CHF)
  ➤ Contraindications
    - Absolute: unstable CHF, severe conduction disease
    - Relative: severe reactive airways disease, COPD
■ Calcium channel blockers (CCBs)
  ➤ Drugs
    - Potent negative inotropic/chronotropic effects: verapamil
    - Mild negative inotropic/chronotropic effects: diltiazem

- Pure vasodilators (dihydropyridines): nifedipine, nicar-dipine, isradipine, nimodipine
➤ Advantages & limitations
  - Verapamil & diltiazem are effective in relieving angina pectoris & decreasing symptom severity & frequency caused by vasospasm (Prinzmetal's angina).
  - Not as effective as beta blockers in decreasing incidence of reinfarction
  - Dihydropyridines are not recommended as they may increase adverse cardiac events.
- Thrombolytic therapy
  ➤ Drugs
    - Streptokinase
    - tPA (tissue plasminogen activator)
    - Reteplase
  ➤ Indications
    - Treatment of acute coronary syndromes
- Heparin
  ➤ Indications
    - In combination w/ aspirin to treat unstable angina
    - After thrombolytic therapy for 3–5 days in AMI
    - For anticoagulation if AF persists >24–36 hrs
    - For anticoagulation when LV thrombus is present
- Warfarin
  ➤ Indications
    - Long-term treatment of unstable angina
    - Combination w/ aspirin more effective than aspirin alone
    - Long-term treatment w/ AF or LV thrombus
- ACE inhibitors
  ➤ Drugs
    - Short acting: captopril
    - Intermediate acting: enalapril (+ IV enalaprilat)
    - Long acting: lisinopril, ramipril

➤ Indications & advantages
- Administered in all pts w/ AMI as BP allows
- Beneficial in pts w/ significant LV dysfunction after AMI (EF < 40%)
- Long-term administration decreases risk of reinfarction & CHF.

➤ Limitations
- Worsened renal function in pts w/ renal insufficiency
- Side effects (eg, cough) may be less w/ angiotensin receptor blockers (ARBs) such as losartan.

■ Lidocaine
➤ Indications
- Only for ventricular dysrhythmias in the setting of AMI

■ Magnesium sulfate
➤ Indications
- Only in pts w/ AMI & torsades de pointes

DRUG DOSING

■ Volatile anesthetics (isoflurane, desflurane & sevoflurane) are safe in the absence of severe CHF.

■ High-dose opioids (50–100 mcg/kg fentanyl) may be used.

■ CAUTION: combination of opioids & nitrous oxide may increase PVR & impair myocardial contractility.

■ Benzodiazepines have minimal cardiovascular effects & are safe to use for anesthetic induction. CAUTION: Higher doses in hypovolemic pts may cause unwanted hypotension.

■ Etomidate may be the drug of choice for induction if severe cardiovascular disease is present, or if any decrease in BP is detrimental.

■ Propofol & thiopental should be used w/ caution because of the risk of hypotension, especially in pts w/ severe IHD & CHF.

■ AVOID sympathomimetic agents (pancuronium, ketamine).

■ CAUTION: CCBs may increase sensitivity to depolarizing & nondepolarizing neuromuscular blocking agents.

LATEX ALLERGY

ARTHUR ATCHABAHIAN, MD

PHARMACOLOGY
Normal

DRUG DOSING
Normal

LIVER DISEASE

ROBERT N. SLADEN, MD

PHARMACOLOGY
- Most IV anesthetic agents are lipid-soluble & non-ionized.
  - Hepatic biotransformation to active or inactive water-soluble metabolites
  - Excreted in bile or urine
- Only lipid-insoluble, highly ionized drugs directly excreted by the kidney
  - Mostly neuromuscular blockers
- Liver disease alters anesthetic & parenteral drug clearance:
  - Decreased blood flow (drug delivery)
  - Increased unbound free fraction of highly protein-bound drugs (hypoalbuminemia, acidosis)
  - Decreased enzymes & transport processes that remove drug from blood
- Mode of biotransformation affects susceptibility to liver injury:
  - Cytochrome CP_{450}: very sensitive (eg, midazolam)
  - Glucuronide conjugation: more robust (eg, lorazepam)
- Pharmacodynamics altered even if pharmacokinetics not changed
  - Pts are debilitated, w/ depleted lean body mass.

➤ Risk of respiratory depression (opioid or volatile anesthetics)
■ Decrease all drug dosages by 25–50%.

DRUG DOSING
■ Drugs independent of renal function for elimination
  ➤ Enzymatic or spontaneous breakdown in the blood
  ➤ Accumulation unlikely
  ➤ Succinylcholine (pseudocholinesterase)
  ➤ Atracurium/cisatracurium (Hofmann elimination)
  ➤ Remifentanil (plasma esterase)
  ➤ Esmolol (RBC esterase)
■ Drugs w/ increased unbound fraction in hypoalbuminemia
  ➤ Increased free or active fraction
  ➤ Decrease doses 20–50% (depending on degree of hypoalbuminemia).
  ➤ Thiopental, methohexital, diazepam
■ Drugs predominantly dependent on hepatic biotransformation
  ➤ Certain volatile agents (>20%: methoxyflurane, halothane)
  ➤ Most perioperative drugs
  ➤ Avoid or decrease dosage in liver failure.
  ➤ All benzodiazepines
  ➤ All opioids
  ➤ Nondepolarizing muscle relaxants (except atracurium, cisatracurium)

MALIGNANT HYPERTHERMIA

HUGH R. PLAYFORD, MD

PHARMACOLOGY
N/A

DRUG DOSING

N/A

MITRAL REGURGITATION

ROBERT N. SLADEN, MD

PHARMACOLOGY

- Chronotropic, inotropic agents are useful.
    - Tachycardia helps maintain CO (fixed stroke volume).
    - Increased contractility compensates for regurgitant fraction.
    - Acute pulmonary hypertension, congestion, edema
- Common maintenance meds & side effects
    - Digoxin (digitoxic conduction disorders, arrhythmias)
    - Loop diuretics (hypokalemia, hyponatremia)
    - Coumadin (bleeding)

DRUG DOSING

N/A

MITRAL STENOSIS

ROBERT N. SLADEN, MD

PHARMACOLOGY

- Avoid chronotropic, inotropic agents.
    - Tachycardia, increased CO increases pressure gradient across mitral valve.
    - Acute pulmonary hypertension, congestion, edema
- Common maintenance meds & side effects
    - Digoxin (digitoxic conduction disorders, arrhythmias)
    - Loop diuretics (hypokalemia, hyponatremia)
    - Coumadin (bleeding)

DRUG DOSING
N/A

MORBID OBESITY

HUGH R. PLAYFORD, MD

PHARMACOLOGY
Changes in pharmacokinetics relate to:
- Increased cardiac output
- Blood volume
- Lean body mass
- Organ size
- Fat mass

Hydrophilic drugs will have relatively normal volume of distribution, elimination half-lives & clearance.

Lipophilic drugs have greater volume of distribution, preferential fat distribution, increased elimination half-life.

Plasma proteins
- Albumin levels unchanged (binding unchanged)
- Alpha-1-glycoprotein increased (increased free fraction basic drugs)
- Triglycerides increased
- Cholesterol increased
- Free fatty acids increased

Pharmacodynamics
- Pseudocholinesterase activity increased
- Increase succinylcholine dose to 1.2–1.5 mg/kg.

Elimination
- Hepatic metabolism
- Phase I metabolism (oxidation, reduction, hydrolysis) unchanged (ie, little change to drugs w/ low intrinsic clearance)
- Phase II metabolism (glucuronidation, sulfation) increased
- High-extraction clearance compound clearance increased

- Renal metabolism
- Glomerular filtration rate increased
- Tubular secretion increased

DRUG DOSING
N/A

MULTIPLE SCLEROSIS

KARL WILLMANN, MD

PHARMACOLOGY

Pharmacotherapy of MS
- Immunomodulation
  - ABC therapy
    - A = Interferon beta 1-a (Avonex)
    - B = Interferon beta 1-b (Betaseron)
    - C = Glatiramer acetate (Copaxone)
  - IVIG (intravenous gamma globulin)
  - Interferon B
    - Antiviral, used when symptoms fluctuate
  - Glatiramer acetate (Copaxone)
    - Used when resistance to interferon B develops
- Immunosuppression
  - Corticosteroids
    - Treats acute symptoms
    - Reduces inflammatory process & length of relapse
  - Azathioprine (Imuran)
  - Methotrexate (Folex)
    - At low doses, inhibits immune responses causing MS
- Anesthetic interactions
  - Benzodiazepines
    - Chronic use may potentiate general anesthetics.
  - Opioids
    - Chronic use leads to tolerance.

➤ Steroids
  - Recent or prolonged use indicates perioperative stress-dose steroid supplementation.
➤ Dantrolene (Dantrium)
  - Increased sensitivity to non-depolarizing muscle relaxants
■ Toxicity
  ➤ Mitoxantrone (Novantrone)
    - Dose-related long-term cardiac toxicity at cumulative doses of 100–140 mg
    - Heart failure & cardiomyopathy have been described at lower doses.
    - Leukopenia, thrombocytopenia
  ➤ Interferon beta 1-a (Avonex)
    - Liver dysfunction & enzyme elevation
    - Anemia, leukopenia, thrombocytopenia
  ➤ Interferon beta 1-b (Betaseron)
    - Liver dysfunction & enzyme elevation
    - Hypertension, leukopenia
  ➤ Glatiramer acetate (Copaxone)
    - Hypertension, eosinophilia
  ➤ IVIG
    - Renal dysfunction & acute renal failure
    - High-dose: hepatitis (nonviral)

DRUG DOSING
N/A

MUSCULAR DYSTROPHY

JONATHAN T. KETZLER, MD

PHARMACOLOGY
■ Succinylcholine may cause rhabdomyolysis, hyperkalemia, malignant hyperthermia & cardiac arrest.
  ➤ Response may occur w/ subclinical disease.

- Nondepolarizing muscle relaxants may result in prolonged paralysis.
- Calcium channel blockers may prolong or even cause neuro-muscular blockade.

DRUG DOSING
N/A

MYASTHENIA GRAVIS

KARL WILLMANN, MD, AND D. B. COURSIN, MD

PHARMACOLOGY
- Pts on anticholinesterases will have prolonged effects w/ both deplorizing & non-depolarizing agents.
- In general, if neuromuscular blockade is needed, then use of nondepolarizing neuromuscular agent would be preferred.
- Depolarizing agents may be unpredictable (resistant, prolonged, normal responses).
  - ➤ MG pt not treated w/ anticholinesterases will be resistant to neuromuscular blockade induced by depolarizing agents.
  - ➤ MG pt treated w/ anticholinesterases (inhibit anticholinesterases) may have prolonged neuromuscular blockade induced by depolarizing agents.
  - ➤ Successive doses of depolarizing agents may induce phase II blockade.
- Pts very sensitive to nondepolarizing agents w/ a high risk of prolonged blockade
- Much interpatient variability of response to neuromuscular blockade
- Atracurium & cis-atracurium are good agents as they have relative short half-lives & do not accumulate w/ repeated doses.
- Must monitor neuromuscular blockade

- Remember that inhalational agents can depress neuromuscular transmission.

DRUG DOSING
- Not all pts require neuromuscular blocking drugs.
- Pts are more susceptible to respiratory decompensation when given narcotics & anxiolytics, which depress respiratory drive.
- Pts are very sensitive to nondepolarizing agents, usually requiring only 10% of the normal dose.
- Pts are usually resistant to depolarizing agents & require 2–3 times the normal dose.
- Consider the supplemental role of inhalational agent depression of neuromuscular transmission.
- Monitor neuromuscular blockade w/ a peripheral nerve stimulator.

NEUROLEPTIC MALIGNANT SYNDROME

HUGH R. PLAYFORD, MD

PHARMACOLOGY
- Unchanged

DRUG DOSING
N/A

OBSTETRIC PATIENT HAVING INTERCURRENT SURGERY

JONATHAN T. KETZLER, MD

PHARMACOLOGY
- Teratogenic effects of anesthetics have not been demonstrated & probably do not exist.

- Nitrous oxide
  - No adverse effect on human pregnancy has been demonstrated.
  - Decreases uterine blood flow in animals
- Benzodiazepines
  - Anecdotal association w/ abnormalities of oral cleft; not substantiated in prospective studies w/ diazepam
- Inhaled agents, IV agents, narcotics & local anesthetics have long history of safety.

DRUG DOSING
- MAC of inhalational anesthetics decreased in the first trimester
- Lower doses of local anesthetics required for equivalent dermatomal spread (epidural venous engorgement & possible increased neural sensitivity)

PARKINSON'S DISEASE

ROBERT N. SLADEN, MD

PHARMACOLOGY
- Disease represents imbalance between CNS dopaminergic & cholinergic transmission.
- Therapy attempts to enhance dopaminergic & block cholinergic transmission.
- Dopaminergic therapy (decreases rigidity, tremor, bradykinesia)
  - L-dopa
  - Carbidopa
  - Bromocriptine
- Anticholinergic therapy (decreases secretions)
  - Atropine

- Pharmacologic considerations relate to side effects & interactions of drug therapy for the disease.

DRUG DOSING
N/A

PATIENT WITH A TRANSPLANT

ARTHUR ATCHABAHIAN, MD

PHARMACOLOGY
- Chronic renal insufficiency
  - Increased extracellular volume
  - Decreased protein binding
  - Decreased elimination of meds dependent on renal function (eg, digoxin, curare, pancuronium)
- Chronic hepatic insufficiency
  - Hypoalbuminemia w/ decreased protein binding
  - Decreased elimination of meds dependent on hepatic function (eg, morphine, vecuronium)

DRUG DOSING
Adjust for renal or hepatic function.

PHEOCHROMOCYTOMA

GIUDITTA ANGELINI, MD

PHARMACOLOGY
- Hypertensive response to histamine, glucagon, droperidol, tyramine, metoclopramide, cytotoxic drugs, saralasin, tricyclic antidepressants, phenothiazines

DRUG DOSING
N/A

PLATELET DISORDERS

KARL WILLMANN, MD

PHARMACOLOGY
- Drugs such as tricyclic antidepressants, chlorpromazine, cocaine, diltiazem, lidocaine, penicillins, cephalosporins & beta blockers may have negative impact on platelet function.
- Drugs such as aspirin, NSAIDs, dipyridamole, ticlopidine, clopidogrel, abciximab & other glycoprotein IIb/IIIa receptor antagonists inhibit normal platelet function.
- Other drugs may affect bone marrow production of platelets, such as thiazides, diuretics, sulfonamides, alcohol.
- Other drugs may potentially mediate immunologically caused platelet destruction, such as heparin, cephalosporins & quinidine.

DRUG DOSING
- No special concerns

POLYCYTHEMIA

KARL WILLMANN, MD, AND DOUGLAS B. COURSIN, MD

PHARMACOLOGY
No specific considerations

DRUG DOSING
- Pts may be receiving hydroxyurea or busulfan to suppress myeloproliferative diseases; interactions w/ these drugs are possible.

PSYCHIATRIC DISORDERS

JONATHAN T. KETZLER, MD

PHARMACOLOGY

- Tricyclic antidepressants
  - Used for treatment of depression & chronic pain
  - All work at nerve synapses to block neuronal reuptake of catecholamines, serotonin or both.
  - Desipramine & nortriptyline most common because fewer side effects & less sedating
  - Amitriptyline, imipramine, protriptyline & doxepin are more sedating.
  - Clomipramine is used to treat obsessive-compulsive disorder.
  - Most have anticholinergic actions
    - Dry mouth, blurred vision, prolonged gastric emptying & urinary retention
    - Amitriptyline has most effect, doxepin has least.
  - Quinidine-like cardiac effects
    - Tachycardia, flattened T waves, PR, QRS & QT prolongation
  - St. John's wort is being used as an OTC antidepressant (see "Herbal Therapy" in the Pharmacology section)
- Monoamine oxidase inhibitors (MAOIs)
  - Block the oxidative deamination of amines
    - MAO A selective for serotonin, dopamine & norepinephrine
    - MAO B selective for tyramine & phenylethylamine
  - Agents available are nonselective MAOIs
  - Side effects include orthostatic hypotension, agitation, tremor, seizures, muscle spasm, urinary retention, paresthesia & jaundice.
  - Hypertensive crisis occurs after ingestion of tyramine-containing foods such as red wine & cheeses.

- Atypical antidepressants
  - ➤ Available agents are primarily selective serotonin reuptake inhibitors
  - ➤ Include fluoxetine, sertraline & paroxetine
  - ➤ Few or no anticholinergic effects
  - ➤ Side effects include headache, agitation & insomnia.

DRUG DOSING
N/A

RESTRICTIVE LUNG DISEASE

HUGH R. PLAYFORD, MBBS

PHARMACOLOGY
Not significantly altered

DRUG DOSING
N/A

RHEUMATOID ARTHRITIS

ROBERT N. SLADEN, MD

PHARMACOLOGY
- Pharmacologic considerations relate to side effects & interactions of drug therapy for the disease.
- Aspirin
  - ➤ Platelet dysfunction (variable, lasts 7–10 days after last dose)
  - ➤ NSAIDs
    - Platelet dysfunction (variable, lasts 24 hrs after last dose)
    - Gastric irritability, erosion (decreased risk with COX-2 inhibitors)

- Nephrotoxicity (not prevented by use of COX-2 inhibitors)
➤ Steroids
  - Adrenal suppression
  - Impaired immune response
  - Peptic ulcer (& increased GI risk w/ NSAIDs)
  - Psychosis
  - Cushing's syndrome (abnormal fat deposition: "moon facies," "buffalo hump")
  - Hypertension
  - Glucose intolerance & frank diabetes
  - Skin fragility (easy bruising, injury)
■ Azothiaprine (Imuran)
  ➤ Bone marrow suppression, immune suppression, liver dysfunction, pancreatitis
■ Cyclophosphamide (Cytoxan)
  ➤ Hemorrhagic cystitis
■ Methotrexate
  ➤ Bone marrow suppression, dermatitis

DRUG DOSING
■ Drugs independent of renal function for elimination
  ➤ Enzymatic or spontaneous breakdown in the blood
    - Accumulation is unlikely
    - Succinylcholine (pseudocholinesterase)
  ➤ Atracurium/cisatracurium (Hofmann elimination)
    - Remifentanil (plasma esterase)
    - Esmolol (RBC esterase)
  ➤ Drugs w/ increased unbound fraction in hypoalbuminemia
    - Increased free or active fraction
    - Decrease doses 20–50% (depending on degree of hypoalbuminemia)
    - Thiopental, methohexital, diazepam

➤ Drugs predominantly dependent on hepatic biotransformation
- Certain volatile agents (>20%: methoxyflurane, halothane)
- Most perioperative drugs
- Avoid or decrease dosage in liver failure.
- All benzodiazepines
- All opioids
- Nondepolarizing muscle relaxants (except atracurium, cisatracurium)

SCLERODERMA

ARTHUR ATCHABAHIAN, MD

PHARMACOLOGY
- Possible renal insufficiency w/ increased extracellular volume & decreased protein binding
- Possible malabsorption w/ hypoproteinemia, leading to increased unbound fraction of protein-bound drugs

DRUG DOSING
- Adjust for renal function.
- Consider following levels for highly protein-bound drugs.
- Use lower doses of opioids because of higher sensitivity.

SICKLE CELL DISEASE

ARTHUR ATCHABAHIAN, MD

PHARMACOLOGY
- Depends on extent of hepatic & renal involvement

DRUG DOSING
- Depends on extent of hepatic & renal involvement

SPINAL CORD INJURY

HUGH R. PLAYFORD, MBBS, AND GEBHARD WAGENER, MD

PHARMACOLOGY

- No significant implications

DRUG DOSING

- No significant implications

STROKE

GEBHARD WAGENER, MD

PHARMACOLOGY

To prevent perioperative stroke:

- Barbiturates reduce cerebral metabolic rate (CMR), but no adequate clinical data for use in acute stroke
- Propofol reduces CMR, cerebral blood flow (CBF) & glutamate release: may reduce infarct size & restore local CBF in ischemic areas
- Inhalational agents: reduce infarct size by redistributing CBF

DRUG DOSING

Pts w/ stroke:

- Avoid succinylcholine w/ significant hemiplegia or hyperkalemia.

If pt is on anti-seizure medication (phenytoin):

- Shortened half-life of non-depolarizing neuromuscular blockers

SUBACUTE BACTERIAL ENDOCARDITIS PROPHYLAXIS

JONATHAN T. KETZLER, MD

PHARMACOLOGY

N/A

DRUG DOSING
- American Heart Association has published recommendations for antibiotic treatment of gram-positive & HACEK endocarditis. However, therapy should always be guided by sensitivity of offending organism.

Dental/Upper Respiratory Tract Surgery
- Low- to medium-risk malformation, no allergy to penicillins
  - ➤ Amoxicillin 3 g orally 1 hr before & 6 hrs after procedure
- High-risk malformation, no allergy to penicillins
  - ➤ Amoxicillin as above or, at physician discretion, ampicillin 1 g IV + gentamicin 1.5 mg/kg IV 0.5 hr before procedure, repeat in 8 hrs if required (or amoxicillin 1.5 g PO)
- Penicillin allergy
  - ➤ Erythromycin 1 g orally 1 hr before & 0.5 g 6 hrs later, or clindamycin 300 mg 1 hr before & 150 mg 6 hrs after procedure, or vancomycin 1 g slowly IV over 1 hr, starting 1 hr before

Genitourinary/Gastrointestinal Procedures
- Oral for low-risk GU/GI procedures, no penicillin allergy
  - ➤ Amoxicillin 3 g orally 1 hr before & 6 hrs after procedure
- Parenteral, no penicillin allergy
  - ➤ Ampicillin 1 g PLUS IV gentamicin 1.5 mg/kg IV 0.5 hr before procedure, repeat both drugs in 8 hrs if required (or amoxicillin 1.5 g PO)
- Penicillin allergy
  - ➤ Vancomycin 1 g slowly IV over 1 hr, starting 1 hr before, PLUS gentamicin 1.5 mg/kg IV, repeat in 8 hrs if required

---

SYSTEMIC LUPUS ERYTHEMATOSUS

ARTHUR ATCHABAHIAN, MD

PHARMACOLOGY
- Possible renal insufficiency w/ increased extracellular volume & decreased protein binding

DRUG DOSING

■ Adjust for renal function.

THALASSEMIA

ARTHUR ATCHABAHIAN, MD

PHARMACOLOGY

■ Depends on extent of hepatic & renal involvement

DRUG DOSING

■ Depends on extent of hepatic & renal involvement

THYROID AND PARATHYROID DISEASE

GIUDITTA ANGELINI, MD

PHARMACOLOGY

■ Hyperthyroidism
  ➤ Thyroxine (T_4) has half-life of 7 days.
  ➤ Tri-iodothyronine (T_3) has half-life of 1.5 days.
  ➤ Carbimazole & propylthiouracil block the synthesis of thyroxine but take 6–8 wks to work.
    • Severe reactions: agranulocytosis, hepatitis, aplastic anemia, lupus-like syndromes
    • Intolerance to these drugs indicates thyroidectomy.
  ➤ Propranolol & other longer-acting beta blockers have been used successfully to treat the symptoms of thyrotoxicosis.
■ Hyperparathyroidism
  ➤ Hypercalcemia enhances digitalis toxicity.

DRUG DOSING

■ Hypothyroidism
  ➤ Impaired drug metabolism

- Hyperthyroidism
  - ➤ Increased clearance & distribution of propofol, may require higher dosage.

TRANSFUSION THERAPY

DOUGLAS B. COURSIN, MD, AND KARL WILLMANN, MD

PHARMACOLOGY
N/A

DRUG DOSING
N/A

VON WILLEBRAND DISEASE

KARL WILLMANN, MD, AND D. B. COURSIN, MD

PHARMACOLOGY
- Avoid drugs that inhibit platelet function.

DRUG DOSING
- No special concerns unless severe liver dysfunction from hepatitis

PART THREE

Clinical Management

ADRENAL & PITUITARY DISEASE

GIUDITTA ANGELINI, MD

SCREENING & EVALUATION

- Basal prolactin concentration
  - Most common adenoma is prolactinoma.
  - >20 ng/mL is abnormal.
  - Differential diagnosis: gonadotroph adenoma (compression), stress
- TSH
  - Primary hypothyroidism can cause pituitary enlargement & secondary compression w/ associated hyperprolactinemia.
  - Hypothyroidism should be treated preop.
  - Primary TSH-secreting adenoma w/ elevated TSH in the setting of elevated thyroid hormones is extremely rare.
- Morning cortisol
  - Compression of sella structures from any adenoma can cause hypopituitarism, which requires investigation of cortisol level.
  - Elevated levels suggest Cushing's syndrome.
  - Cortisol level maintained w/ dexamethasone suppression test except pituitary Cushing's, which may suppress w/ high dose
- Measure ACTH concentration under dexamethasone suppression.
  - Undetectable level: adrenal tumor
  - 10–100 ng/L: pituitary-dependent tumor
  - >200 ng/L: ectopic ACTH secretion
  - Selective petrosal sinus sampling of ACTH after CRH stimulation can confirm pituitary Cushing's syndrome.
- Growth hormone concentration
  - Random >5 ng/mL: abnormal

➤ Failure to suppress to <1 ng/mL following 75-g glucose load: diagnostic
■ MRI is superior to CT for imaging the pituitary.

PREOPERATIVE PREPARATION
■ Assess visual function (visual field defects, third cranial nerve).
■ Assess for signs & symptoms of increased ICP.
■ Acromegaly
  ➤ Assess macroglossia & thickening of pharyngeal tissues, thickened vocal cords, reduction in laryngeal aperture: difficult airway
  ➤ 25% have enlarged thyroid, which may compress trachea.
  ➤ Thickened periepiglottic folds may result in recurrent laryngeal nerve palsy.
  ➤ Sleep apnea may be severe; respiratory failure is threefold higher in this population.
  ➤ Assess treatment of hypertension & glucose intolerance.
■ Cushing's syndrome
  ➤ Assess mgt of hypertension & glucose intolerance.
  ➤ 18% have severe sleep apnea.
  ➤ Anticipate gastroesophageal reflux disease.
  ➤ Anticipate suppressed immune system.
  ➤ Fragile skin makes IV access problematic.

OPERATIVE PREPARATION
■ Transsphenoidal approach is used most commonly (fewer postop complications than sublabial or endonasal approach).
  ➤ Lower risk of postop seizures
  ➤ Minimal risk of trauma or hemorrhage
  ➤ Less likely for total ablation of pituitary & postop need for hormone replacement
■ Transcranial approach: large tumor, small/non-pneumatized sphenoid sinus

ANESTHESIA

- Continue preop hormone replacement during operative period, w/ hydrocortisone on the day of surgery.
- Airway mgt in acromegalics will require large masks & longer blades.
    - ➤ Ventilation w/ bag & mask is generally straightforward w/ an oral airway.
    - ➤ Pts w/ glottic stenosis & vocal cord paresis, especially w/ pharyngeal mucosal hypertrophy, are likely to require fiberoptic intubation.
    - ➤ Intubating laryngeal mask airway has been used successfully.
    - ➤ Equipment for tracheostomy should be available.
- Cocaine used for nasal vasoconstriction has been associated w/ arrhythmias & MI.
    - ➤ Xylometazoline is an alpha agonist that when combined w/ lidocaine can be equivalent to cocaine.
- Lumbar drains may be placed.
    - ➤ 10-mL aliquots of 0.9% saline can be introduced to produce prolapse of suprasellar portion of tumor into operative field.
    - ➤ Should the dura be breached during surgery, the catheter can be left in place to control CSF leak.
- Pt will be positioned supine w/ head-up tilt; surgeon will be at head of table or just to the right or left, so appropriate secured airway approach is necessary.
- Inhalation or IV anesthetic is equivalent, but avoid nitrous oxide in pts w/ increased ICP.
- Short-acting agents are important to allow for quick emergence & neurologic assessment.
- Excessive hyperventilation may make suprasellar extension less accessible.
- Most stimulating period is during transsphenoidal access.
- Bilateral maxillary block has been successful for transsphenoidal approach.

- Standard ASA monitors
  - Comorbidities may require more invasive monitoring, especially in Cushing's pts.
  - If a steep head-up tilt is used, monitoring for venous air embolism may be required.
  - Visual evoked potentials have a high incidence of false negatives & false positives in the OR & are easily interfered w/ by anesthetic agents.
- Cefuroxime is recommended for prophylaxis preop.
- Transsphenoidal approach has rare complications of carotid or pons disruption.
- Transcranial approach has rare complications of frontal lobe ischemia, trauma to carotid or optic chiasm & anosmia secondary to damage to olfactory tract.

WAKE UP & EMERGENCE
- Smooth & rapid emergence is essential.
- May have throat pack to remove & nasal packs, which need to stay in place

ICU OR PACU
- Usually only transcranial approach requires ICU.
- Given nasal packs, all pts w/ transsphenoidal surgery must be fully awake postop before being moved to general floor, since CPAP is relatively difficult to administer.
- Transcranial approach will require more opioid analgesia.
- Endocrinologist: continued hormone replacement
- Hydrocortisone is usually imperative in most cases in which it has been used preop.
  - Prolactinomas w/ >20% of pituitary remaining likely can be quickly reduced.
  - Pts w/ Cushing's syndrome likely will require slower weaning over wks.
- Diabetes insipidus
  - Occurs when >80% of neurons synthesizing vasopressin are destroyed

- ➤ >1 L of dilute urine in 12 hrs (<300 mOsmol/kg)
- ➤ Plasma sodium concentration >143 mmol/L
- ➤ Plasma osmolality >295 mOsmol/kg
- ➤ Awake pts should be allowed free access to fluid.
- ➤ DDAVP may be administered 0.04–0.1 mcg 1–3 times daily; can also be administered intranasally.
- ■ Hyponatremia can be related to excessive DDAVP or SIADH
  - ➤ Fluid restriction is indicated for transitory SIADH secondary to pituitary disruption.
  - ➤ Cerebral salt wasting w/ natriuresis & diuresis requires administration of hypertonic saline over 24–48 hrs.
  - ➤ Rapid replacement will result in central pontine myelinolysis.
- ■ Bilateral adrenalectomy surgery for ACTH tumors requires mineralocorticoid & glucocorticoid supplementation.
  - ➤ Carries risk of Nelson's syndrome w/ hyperpigmentation & compression of parapituitary structures secondary to melanocyte-stimulating hormone
- ■ Vocal cord changes in acromegaly mostly resolve after 10 days.
- ■ While left ventricular size may normalize after surgery in pts w/ acromegaly, interstitial myocardial fibrosis does not resolve & left ventricular dysfunction persists.

ADULT CONGENITAL HEART DISEASE

MARY E. McSWEENEY, MD

SCREENING & EVALUATION

Studies

- ■ Review echo & cath studies to determine anatomy, blood flow characteristics & ventricular function.

  Note whether elevated PVR is reversible.

- EKG (heart block, ischemic changes, arrhythmia, ventricular & atrial enlargement)
- Chest x-ray: anatomy, CHF, diaphragmatic paresis, atelectasis
- Labs (elevated Hct & platelets commonly associated w/ hypoxic lesions; platelet function often abnormal & clotting factors often reduced)

Physical exam
- Hypoxemia: clubbing of nails, cyanosis
- Ventricular hypertrophy (apical heave)
- Congestive heart failure (elevated neck veins, edema, hepatomegaly)

PREOPERATIVE PREPARATION
- No contraindication to preop sedation in adults w/ CHD; pts w/ high PVR generally benefit from anxiolysis as long as hypoventilation is avoided
- Diuretics are usually held the morning of surgery to ensure adequate intravascular volume.
- Antibiotics for prevention of bacterial endocarditis are required for all but the most benign of CHD lesions (such as pts status post primary repair of ASD or VSD) in cases w/ any potential for bacterial seeding.
- Use air filters in venous lines for any pt w/ possibility of R-to-L shunting.

OPERATIVE PREPARATION
N/A

ANESTHESIA
- Pts w/ severe pulmonary hypertension can be high risk w/ both general & regional anesthesia. Nerve blocks are preferable to general, spinal or epidural anesthesia when possible.
  - ➤ Fixed PVR is unresponsive to pharmacologic treatment.

➤ Avoid factors known to increase PVR: hypothermia, acidosis, hypercarbia, hypoxia & endogenous or exogenous catecholamines w/ alpha-adrenergic effects.

➤ Hypovolemia & systemic vasodilation both increase R-to-L shunt.

■ Volatile anesthetics are tolerated well in most pts w/ CHD.

➤ Negative chronotropic & inotropic actions are dose-dependent.

■ Nitrous oxide

➤ May be used to supplement volatile anesthetics for induction.

➤ Avoid for maintenance (increased PVR, intravascular bubble enlargement).

■ Vascular access can be complicated by anatomy or previous surgical procedures

➤ Femoral vein thrombosis or ligation

➤ Discontinuity of IVC & RA

➤ Reduced lower extremity BP w/ coarctation

➤ Discontinuity of subclavian artery w/ BT anastomosis

➤ Artifactually elevated right arm BP w/ supravalvular aortic stenosis

WAKE UP & EMERGENCE

■ Avoid coughing & straining on extubation; can worsen R-to-L shunt.

■ General anesthesia & intubation

Consider gradual wake up & extubation in ICU.

ICU OR PACU

■ Optimize pain control to minimize straining, which can worsen R-to-L shunt.

■ ICU care strongly recommended postop for any pt w/ complex or cyanotic CHD recovering from anesthesia & surgery

ALCOHOL ABUSE

JONATHAN T. KETZLER, MD

SCREENING & EVALUATION

- Screening strategies to identify pts w/ alcohol abuse
  - Physical findings
    - Rhinophyma, telangiectasias
    - Tremulousness, unexplained tachycardia, elevated BP
    - Unexplained hepatosplenomegaly, peripheral neuropathy
    - Unexplained physical trauma.
  - Physical exam may be completely normal.
- Evaluate end-organ damage.
  - Macrocytosis (MCV 100–110 fL): 90% of cases, precedes overt anemia
  - Elevated liver enzymes (AST, ALT, GGT)
  - Alcoholic hepatitis: AST $\gg$ ALT (>2.0) is highly specific.
    - Serum carbohydrate-deficient transferrin (CDT): approved by FDA as indicator of chronic heavy alcohol consumption (sensitivity 60–70%, specificity 80–90%)
- Prompt intervention prior to surgery

PREOPERATIVE PREPARATION

- Abstinence (at least 1 month)
  - Decreases risk of postop complications
- Detoxification (depends on patient motivation, urgency of surgery)

OPERATIVE PREPARATION

- Prophylaxis of alcohol withdrawal
  - Decreased risk of postop complications & prolonged ICU stay.

➤ Benzodiazepines (diazepam, lorazepam or chlordiazepoxide)

ANESTHESIA

- Anticipate larger dose requirement for induction of action (increased volume of distribution).
  ➤ Eg, propofol, fentanyl, pancuronium
- Alcoholics require significantly larger doses of fentanyl than nondrinkers to achieve adequate analgesia at the time of surgery.
- Acute alcohol consumption: Anticipate prolonged duration of some drug action (eg, propranolol, phenobarbital).
- Chronic alcohol consumption: Anticipate shortened duration of some drug action (induction of cytochrome P450 system).
- Anticipate increased sympathetic & cortisol response to surgical stress; immunosuppression & increased postop morbidity.
- Surgical stress response can mimic, precipitate & exacerbate alcohol withdrawal syndromes.

Intraoperative hypoxemia or hypotension increases risk of postop delirium.

WAKE UP & EMERGENCE
N/A

ICU OR PACU

- Increased risk of postop:
  ➤ Arrhythmias (without overt cardiac disease).
    • "Holiday heart syndrome" (binge drinking)
  ➤ Bleeding
  ➤ Surgical site infections
  ➤ Impaired wound healing
  ➤ Prolonged intubation & ICU stay

ANEMIA AND HEMOGLOBINOPATHIES

DOUGLAS B. COURSIN, MD AND KARL WILLMANN, MD

SCREENING AND EVALUATION

- CBC, Hgb not routinely acquired for most outpatients & many inpatients
- Identify high-risk pts (+ active or known history of anemia)
  - Obtain CBC
    - Determines WBC, Hct, Hgb, platelet count & indices
    - Reticulocyte count: bone marrow activity

PREOPERATIVE PREPARATION

- Identify anemia in high-risk pts or those undergoing high-risk surgery.
- Determine if anemia is of physiologic importance.
- Determine etiology:
  - Acute or chronic: Compensated or not?
  - If blood loss: Is it controlled? Does procedure need to be performed to control bleeding?
  - If secondary to nutrient deficiency: Does pt require supplementation (iron, vitamin B12, folate)? Is pt at risk for associated pathology? Neurologic disease w/ vitamin B12 deficiency? Abnormal homocysteine metabolism & folate?
  - Would the pt benefit from perioperative EPO?
    - Facilitate autologous predonation
    - Augment perioperative treatment of anemia
    - Available drugs: human recombinant EPO, darbopoietin
- Transfusion therapy
  - Based on acuity and severity of anemia, associated pathology, risk of surgery/procedure

OPERATIVE PREPARATION

- Address need for transfusion.
- Type & screen or cross-match if needed & not already performed.
- Determine availability of blood preop.

ANESTHESIA

- Maintain O_2 delivery.
  - Correct hypovolemia.
  - Avoid meds that depress cardiac function.
  - Avoid left shift in O_2 dissociation curve:
    - Avoid hypothermia (but may provide CNS protection).
    - Avoid acute alkalosis.
  - Avoid N_2O in pts w/ vitamin B12 or folate deficiencies.
  - "Transfusion trigger" based on level of anemia, anticipated blood loss, individual reserve

WAKE UP AND EMERGENCE

- Maintain O_2 delivery by maintaining good circulatory status
- Treat shivering, excessive tachycardia or hypertension.

ICU OR PACU

- >50% of ICU pts are anemic within 72 hrs of ICU admission.
- 1/7 ICU pts per day receive a transfusion in the ICU.
- Over a third of all ICU pts receive transfusion during their ICU course.
- Risk of transfusion increases with length of ICU stay.
- Transfusions are independently associated w/ increased length of ICU stay, morbidity & mortality.
- Increase transfusion trigger: CNS injury, myocardial ischemia or infarction

ANKYLOSING SPONDYLITIS

HUGH R. PLAYFORD, MD

SCREENING AND EVALUATION

- Note the following:
  - ➤ Previous anesthesia (difficulty w/ intubation, nerve blocks, positioning)
  - ➤ Spinal fracture
  - ➤ Spinal surgery
  - ➤ Medications (NSAIDs, corticosteroids, phenylbutazone, sulfasalazine, azathioprine, methotrexate, cyclophosphamide)
- Look for physical signs of:
  - ➤ CHF, arrhythmia, uveitis, upper & lower motor nerve signs
  - ➤ Limited mouth opening, vocal abnormality, limited neck movement, neck pain
- Relevant lab studies
  - ➤ Hct, CBC
  - ➤ ABGs on room air
  - ➤ ECG, chest x-ray
  - ➤ W/ or w/out echo
  - ➤ PFTs (usually restrictive pattern w/ slight to moderate decreased in VC & TLC, normal to increased FRC & VC, normal airflow rates, decreased maximal expiratory & inspiratory pressures)
  - ➤ Cervical spine x-ray (w/ flexion-extension)

PREOPERATIVE PREPARATION

- Airway evaluation (w/ or w/out ENT laryngeal assessment)
- W/ or w/out preparation for awake fiberoptic nasopharyngeal intubation
- Pulmonary function assessment

- Positioning considerations
- Minimize sedative or opioid premeds.
- Neurologic exam for upper & lower motor nerve deficits.
- Analgesic considerations intraop & postop (avoid respiratory depressants)

OPERATIVE PREPARATION

- Minimize sedative or opioid premeds.
- Use universal & aseptic precautions throughout.
- Difficult airway preparation
  - ➤ Antisialagogue
  - ➤ Nasal preparation
  - ➤ Difficult airway cart (including fiberoptic bronchoscope)
- Invasive hemodynamic monitoring if:
  - ➤ Cardiopulmonary insufficiency
  - ➤ Large fluid shifts anticipated
- Care w/ positioning, pad pressure points

ANESTHESIA

- Regional anesthesia
  - ➤ Not contraindicated
  - ➤ Document any neurologic deficits preop.
  - ➤ Skeletal abnormality may make regional block technically difficult & response to local anesthetic unpredictable.
- General anesthesia
  - ➤ Consider positioning difficulties (including perioperative spinal fracture).
  - ➤ Potential for difficult airway
  - ➤ Preoxygenation (limited respiratory reserve)
  - ➤ Avoid myocardial depressants if limited cardiac reserve.
  - ➤ Low pulmonary compliance but usually normal lung compliance

WAKE UP AND EMERGENCE

- Avoid excessive sedation.

- Optimize analgesia w/out respiratory depression.
- Extubate when fully awake.

ICU OR PACU
- Careful respiratory monitoring

ANTICOAGULATION THERAPY

JONATHAN T. KETZLER, MD

SCREENING AND EVALUATION
N/A

PREOPERATIVE PREPARATION
N/A

OPERATIVE PREPARATION
N/A

ANESTHESIA
- Anesthetic mgt of the pt receiving thrombolytic therapy
  - Thrombolytic drugs should be avoided for 10 days following the puncture of noncompressible vessels.
    - Ideally this would include lumbar puncture, neuraxial anesthesia & epidural steroid injection.
  - It should be determined preoperatively whether fibrinolytic or thrombolytic drugs have been used preoperatively or might be used intraoperatively or postoperatively. There are no clear data to suggest how long neuraxial anesthesia should be avoided after the use of these drugs.
  - Pts who do receive neuraxial anesthesia at or near the time of treatment w/ fibrinolytic or thrombolytic drugs should have their neurologic status monitored at intervals of no more than 2 hrs.

- If pt has a neuraxial catheter in place, avoid drugs that might interfere w/ neurologic exam.
➤ Although there are no recommendations for timing of the removal of a neuraxial catheter after the use of fibrinolytic or thrombolytic drugs, the measurement of fibrinogen (one of the last clotting factors to recover) may be helpful.
- Anesthetic mgt of the pt receiving unfractionated heparin
  ➤ There are no contraindications to the use of neuraxial anesthesia in the pt receiving subcutaneous (mini-dose) heparin.
    - Delaying the injection until after the block may reduce the risk of neuraxial bleeding.
    - Prolonged therapy in debilitated pts may increase the risk of neuraxial bleeding.
    - Pts receiving heparin for >4 days should have a platelet count because of the risk of heparin-induced thrombocytopenia.
  ➤ Intraoperative anticoagulation can be combined w/ neuraxial anesthesia, w/ the following cautions:
    - Avoid neuraxial anesthesia in pts w/ other coagulopathies.
    - Delay anticoagulation w/ heparin for 1 hr after placement of the needle.
    - Remove indwelling neuraxial catheters 2–4 hrs after the last heparin dose, after the pt's coagulation status has been evaluated.
      - Delay re-heparinization until 1 hr after the catheter has been removed.
    - The pt should be monitored postoperatively for early detection of motor blockade. Minimal concentration of local anesthetics should be used for better detection of spinal hematoma.

- There are no data to suggest that a bloody or difficult neuraxial needle placement should require cancellation of the case. Discuss the specific risks & benefits of continuing w/ the surgeon.

➤ There are insufficient data to determine whether there is an increased risk of neuraxial hematoma if neuraxial anesthesia is combined w/ the full anticoagulation of cardiac surgery.

- The pt should be monitored postoperatively for early detection of motor blockade. Minimal concentration of local anesthetics should be used for better detection of spinal hematoma.
- The concurrent use of meds that also affect the clotting cascade, such as antiplatelet therapy, low-molecular-weight heparin (LMWH) & oral anticoagulants, may increase the risk of neuraxial hematoma.

■ Anesthetic mgt of the pt receiving low-molecular-weight heparin (LMWH)

➤ These recommendations were developed using the extensive experience of European anesthesiologists w/ LMWH.

- The level of anti-Xa is not predictive of the risk of bleeding, so it is not helpful in the mgt of pts undergoing neuraxial anesthesia.
- The concurrent use of meds that also affect the clotting cascade, such as antiplatelet therapy, unfractionated heparin & oral anticoagulants, may increase the risk of neuraxial hematoma.
- Delay the initiation of LMWH for 24 hrs postoperatively if there is the presence of blood during needle placement.
- Traumatic needle or catheter placement may cause an increased risk of neuraxial hematoma; discuss the specific risks & benefits of continuing w/ the surgeon.

- Preop LMWH
  - Pts on LMWH preoperatively should be assumed to have altered coagulation, so delay placement of a needle until 10–12 hrs after the last dose of LMWH.
  - In pts on higher-than-prophylactic doses, such as enoxaparin 1 mg/kg q12h, enoxaparin 1.5 mg/kg daily, dalteparin 120 U/kg q12h, dalteparin 200 U/kg daily or tinzaparin 175 U/kg daily, delay placement of the needle at least 24 hrs.
  - Avoid neuraxial techniques in pts who have received LMWH 2 hours before, because this is the peak of anticoagulant activity.
- Postop LMWH
  - Mgt of pts receiving postop LMWH is based on total dose, timing of first postop dose & dosing schedule.
  - Twice-daily dosing may be associated w/ an increased risk of neuraxial hematoma.
    - Regardless of anesthetic technique, give the first dose no sooner than 24 hours postop, & only in the setting of adequate surgical hemostasis.
    - Continuous catheters may be left in overnight & removed the next morning 2 hrs prior to the first dose.
  - Single daily dose approximates the European application.
  - Give the first post dose 6–8 hrs postop.
  - The second dose should not be given sooner than 24 hrs after the first dose.
  - Neuraxial catheters may be left indwelling & should be removed no sooner than 10–12 hrs after the last dose of LMWH.
  - Subsequent dosing should occur no sooner than 2 hrs after catheter removal.

- Regional anesthetic mgt of the patient on oral anticoagulants
  - ➤ These recommendations are based on warfarin pharmacology, the clinical relevance of vitamin K coagulation factor levels/deficiencies & case reports of spinal hematomas.
  - ➤ Stop oral anticoagulation 4–5 days prior to planned procedure.
    - Early after discontinuation of warfarin therapy, the PT/INR reflects predominantly factor VII levels; however, levels of factors II, VII, IX & X may not be adequate until 5–7 days.
    - The concurrent use of meds that also affect the clotting cascade, such as antiplatelet therapy, unfractionated heparin & LMWH, may increase the risk of neuraxial hematoma without affecting the PT/INR.
    - For pts receiving a preop dose of oral anticoagulants, check PT/INR before placement of neuraxial anesthesia if the dose was given >24 hours prior or if a second dose has been given.
    - For pts who receive low-dose warfarin therapy during epidural analgesia, monitor PT/INR daily & before catheter removal.
      - Studies evaluating the use of warfarin w/ epidural analgesia used daily doses of 5 mg warfarin. Higher doses require more intensive monitoring of coagulation studies.
    - When thromboprophylaxis is initiated w/ warfarin, remove the catheter while the INR is <1.5.
    - In pts w/ indwelling neuraxial catheters, withhold warfarin if the INR is >3.0.
      - There are no recommendations for removal of a neuraxial catheter in pts w/ therapeutic levels of anticoagulation.

- Use lower doses of warfarin in pts who are likely to have an enhanced response to the drug.
- Anesthetic mgt of the pt receiving antiplatelet meds
  - ➤ Antiplatelet meds include NSAIDs, thienopyridine derivatives (ticlopidine, clopidogrel) & platelet GP IIb/IIIa antagonists (abciximab, eptifibatide, tirofiban). They exert diverse effects on platelet function.
  - ➤ There is no way to extrapolate btwn groups of drugs regarding neuraxial anesthesia.
  - ➤ No test, including bleeding time, adequately assesses antiplatelet therapy.
    - Careful preop assessment of a history of easy bruising or bleeding, female gender & increased age should be used to make decisions regarding neuraxial anesthesia.
  - ➤ The use of NSAIDs alone should not interfere w/ the performance of neuraxial anesthesia.
    - This includes timing of single shot or catheter techniques, postop monitoring & timing of catheter removal.
  - ➤ The risk of spinal hematoma w/ ticlopidine & clopidogrel & the GP IIb/IIIa antagonists is not known.
  - ➤ Recommendations are based on labeling precautions & the surgical, interventional cardiology/radiology experience.
    - Based on labeling & surgical reviews, the suggested time interval btwn discontinuation of thienopyridine therapy & neuraxial blockade is 14 days for ticlopidine, 7 days for clopidogrel.
    - Platelet GP IIb/IIIa inhibitors exert a profound effect on platelet function.
    - Following administration, the time to normal platelet aggregation is 24–48 hrs for abciximab, 4–8 hrs for eptifibatide & tirofiban.

- Avoid neuraxial techniques until platelet function has recovered.
- GP IIb/IIIa antagonists are contraindicated within 4 wks of surgery.
- If a GP IIb/IIIa antagonist is administered in the postop period (following a neuraxial technique), the pt should be carefully monitored neurologically.

➤ The concurrent use of other meds affecting clotting mechanisms, such as oral anticoagulants, unfractionated heparin & LMWH, may increase the risk of bleeding complications.

➤ Cyclooxygenase-2 inhibitors have a minimal effect on platelet function & should be considered in pts who require anti-inflammatory therapy in the presence of anti-coagulation.

■ Anesthetic mgt of the patient receiving herbal therapy

➤ A significant number of surgical pts use alternative meds.

➤ There is no evidence that herbal therapy represents an added risk for development of neuraxial hematoma.

➤ There is no evidence that neuraxial anesthesia should be avoided or surgery cancelled if the pt has used herbal therapies.

➤ There are no data on the concurrent use of other forms of anticoagulation w/ herbal therapies.

- Concurrent use of other forms of anticoagulation w/ herbal therapy may increase the risk of neuraxial hematoma.

➤ There is no test to assess the adequacy of hemostasis in pts using herbal meds.

➤ The use of herbal medicine alone should not interfere w/ the performance of neuraxial anesthesia.

- This includes timing of single shot or catheter techniques, postop monitoring or the timing of catheter removal.
- New anticoagulants (direct thrombin inhibitors and fondaparinux)
  - New antithrombotic drugs target various steps in the hemostatic system, such as inhibiting platelet aggregation, blocking coagulation factors or enhancing fibrinolysis.
  - The most extensively studied are antagonists of specific platelet receptors & direct thrombin inhibitors.
  - Many of these antithrombotic agents have prolonged half-lives & are difficult to reverse w/out the administration of blood components.
  - Thrombin inhibitors
    - Recombinant hirudin derivatives include desirudin, lepirudin, bivalirudin.
      - Recombinant hirudin derivatives inhibit both free & clot-bound thrombin.
    - Argatroban, an L-arginine derivative, has a similar mechanism of action.
    - There are no case reports of spinal hematoma related to neuraxial anesthesia among pts who have received a thrombin inhibitor.
      - Spontaneous intracranial bleeding has been reported.
    - There are no recommendations regarding risk assessment & pt mgt.
    - Identification of interventional cardiac & surgical risk factors associated w/ bleeding after invasive procedures may be helpful.
  - Fondaparinux
    - Fondaparinux produces its antithrombotic effect through factor Xa inhibition.

- The FDA released fondaparinux with a black box warning similar to that of the LMWHs & heparinoids.
- The actual risk of spinal hematoma with fondaparinux is unknown.
- Until further clinical experience is available, performance of neuraxial techniques should occur under conditions used in clinical trials (single needle pass, atraumatic needle placement, avoidance of indwelling neuraxial catheters).

■ Summary

➤ The consensus paper concludes by stating:

➤ "Practice guidelines or recommendations summarize evidence-based reviews. However, the rarity of spinal hematoma defies a prospective-randomized study, and there is no current laboratory model. As a result, these consensus statements represent the collective experience of recognized experts in the field of neuraxial anesthesia and anticoagulation. They are based on case reports, clinical series, pharmacology, hematology, and risk factors for surgical bleeding. An understanding of the complexity of this issue is essential to patient management; a cookbook approach is not appropriate. Rather, the decision to perform spinal or epidural anesthesia/analgesia and the timing of catheter removal in a patient receiving antithrombotic therapy should be made on an individual basis, weighing the small, though definite risk of spinal hematoma with the benefits of regional anesthesia for a specific patient. Alternative anesthetic and analgesic techniques exist for patients considered an unacceptable risk. The patient's coagulation status should be optimized at the time of spinal or epidural needle/catheter placement, and the level of anticoagulation must be carefully monitored during the period of epidural catheterization. Indwelling catheters should not be removed in the presence of therapeutic anticoagulation, as this appears to significantly increase the risk of spinal hematoma. It must also be remembered that identification of risk factors and establishment of guidelines will not completely eliminate the complication of spinal hematoma. Vigilance in monitoring is critical to allow early evaluation of neurologic dysfunction and prompt intervention. We must focus not only on the prevention of spinal hematoma, but also optimization of neurologic outcome."

WAKE UP AND EMERGENCE
N/A

ICU OR PACU
N/A

AORTIC REGURGITATION

ROBERT N. SLADEN, MD

SCREENING AND EVALUATION
- Note the following:
  - ➤ Symptoms (dyspnea, syncope, congestive heart failure)
  - ➤ Signs of progressive disease (pulse pressure, ECG changes, cardiomegaly, degree of AR)
  - ➤ Presence of associated CAD (increased risk)
- Look for physical signs of:
  - ➤ LVH (apical heave)
  - ➤ Congestive heart failure (elevated neck veins, edema, hepatomegaly)
- Relevant lab studies
  - ➤ Hct (anemia is poorly tolerated by low CO)

- PT, INR (if on coumadin for atrial fib)
- BUN, creatinine (prerenal syndrome)
- ECG (LVH w/ or w/out strain)
- Chest x-ray (LVH)
- TTE, TEE (AR, LVH, LAH)

PREOPERATIVE PREPARATION

- Continue preop meds:
  - Digoxin (inotropy, rate control for atrial fib)
  - Diuretics for pulmonary edema
- Plan perioperative anticoagulation:
  - Hold coumadin at least 3 days preop.
  - Check INR prior to surgery.
- Consider preop admission for control of:
  - Rapid atrial fib
  - Symptomatic pulmonary edema or congestive heart failure
- Plan perioperative antibiotics:
  - Increased risk of bacterial endocarditis

OPERATIVE PREPARATION

- Review hemodynamic principles:
  - Maintain sinus rhythm (atrial kick, to maximize ventricular filling)
  - Maintain faster heart rate (decrease diastolic regurgitant time)
  - Maintain adequate preload (maximize ventricular filling)
  - Use inotropic, chronotropic agents (maintain contractility, heart rate)
  - Dopamine (beta-adrenergic dose range)
  - Dobutamine (inodilator, provides afterload reduction)
  - Avoid systemic vasoconstrictors.
- Acute (new-onset) atrial fib

- ➤ Poorly tolerated, can induce acute decompensation, low cardiac output syndrome
- ➤ Treat aggressively whenever it occurs (esmolol, amiodarone, early cardioversion).
- ■ Avoid excessive sedative or opioid premed:
  - ➤ Suppresses catecholamines, induces bradycardia
  - ➤ Increased risk of respiratory depression (hypercarbia increases PVR)
- ■ Use fluids & inotropic + chronotropic agents to treat hypotension:
  - ➤ Maintain preload, diastolic perfusion pressure.
  - ➤ Use ephedrine (mixed agonist, increases contractility, may induce tachycardia).
  - ➤ Avoid vasoconstrictors (phenylephrine, norepinephrine): increase SVR
- ■ Invasive hemodynamic monitoring, TEE
  - ➤ Moderate to large fluid shifts anticipated
  - ➤ Presence of symptoms

ANESTHESIA
- ■ Regional anesthesia is relatively contraindicated:
  - ➤ Sympathetic block may induce dangerous hypotension, worsen MVO_2
  - ➤ Avoid spinal anesthesia (abrupt onset of block)
  - ➤ Careful continuous spinal or epidural anesthesia may be tolerated
  - ➤ Adequate fluid load prior to placement (maintain preload)
- ■ General anesthesia
  - ➤ Take measures to maintain faster heart rate & adequate contractility
  - ➤ Preoxygenate
  - ➤ Adequate fluid load prior to induction (maintain preload)
  - ➤ Treat hypotension w/ ephedrine
  - ➤ Treat bradycardia w/ ephedrine, dopamine, dobutamine

- Choose maintenance regimen that maintains faster heart rate, avoids myocardial depression:
  - Consider low-dose isoflurane (increased heart rate), desflurane (increased sympathetic tone).
  - Consider total IV anesthetic (fentanyl, sufentanil, remifentanil), but watch for bradycardia.

WAKE UP AND EMERGENCE

- Attempt to suppress catecholamines on emergence (tachyarrhythmias)
  - Judicious use of sympatholytic opioid (fentanyl, sufentanil, remifentanil)
  - Avoid morphine (histamine, catecholamine release)
- Potential complications on emergence
  - Delayed emergence (low cardiac output, increased pharmacodynamic effects)
  - Acute pulmonary hypertension
  - Acute pulmonary congestion, edema
  - Hypoxemia, acute respiratory failure

ICU OR PACU

- Maintain cardiac output
  - Maintain preload (fluids)
  - Aggressive treatment of atrial arrhythmias (esmolol, amiodarone, cardioversion)
  - Maintain or increase contractility (dopamine)
    - Decrease afterload with vasodilators (nitroprusside, nicardipine)
    - Increase contractility, decrease afterload with inodilators (dobutamine, milrinone)
- Consider short period of postop mechanical ventilation if AR severe:
  - Allows controlled emergence
  - Avoids reversal (ie, need for muscarinic agents [bradycardia])

> Facilitates evaluation of cardiac, ventilatory function
> Allows control of pulmonary hypertension, appropriate diuresis prior to extubation
- Restart preop meds (digoxin, diuretics) as soon as possible.
- For chronic atrial fib:
  > Anticoagulation required >24 hrs to prevent intracardiac thrombus formation
  > Restart oral coumadin when pt is able to take orally.
  > If not, start IV heparin & continue until pt is able to take oral meds.

AORTIC STENOSIS

ROBERT N. SLADEN, MD

SCREENING AND EVALUATION
- Note the following:
  > Symptoms (angina, syncope, congestive heart failure)
  > Signs of progressive disease (ECG changes, valve gradient & area)
  > Presence of associated CAD (increased risk)
- Look for physical signs of:
  > Left ventricular hypertrophy (apical heave)
  > Congestive heart failure (elevated neck veins, edema, hepatomegaly)
- Relevant lab studies
  > Hct (anemia is poorly tolerated by low CO)
  > PT, INR (if on coumadin for AF)
  > BUN, creatinine (prerenal syndrome)
  > ECG (LVH w/ or w/out strain)
  > Chest x-ray (LVH)

PREOPERATIVE PREPARATION
- Continue preop meds:
  > Beta blockade or calcium blockade (negative inotropy, chronotropy)

- ➤ Digoxin (rate control for atrial fibrillation)
- ➤ Diuretics for pulmonary edema
- ■ Plan perioperative anticoagulation
  - ➤ Hold coumadin at least 3 days preoperatively.
  - ➤ Check INR before surgery.
- ■ Consider preop admission for control of:
  - ➤ Rapid atrial fibrillation
  - ➤ Symptomatic pulmonary edema or congestive heart failure
- ■ Plan perioperative antibiotics:
  - ➤ Decrease risk of bacterial endocarditis

OPERATIVE PREPARATION
- ■ Review hemodynamic principles
  - ➤ Maintain sinus rhythm (atrial kick, to maximize ventricular filling).
  - ➤ Maintain slow heart rate (increase diastolic fill time).
  - ➤ Maintain adequate preload (maximize ventricular filling).
  - ➤ Avoid inotropic, chronotropic agents.
  - ➤ Avoid systemic vasodilators.
  - ➤ Maintain SVR (& coronary diastolic perfusion pressure).
- ■ Acute (new-onset) atrial fibrillation
  - ➤ Poorly tolerated; can induce acute decompensation, low cardiac output syndrome
  - ➤ Treat aggressively whenever it occurs (esmolol, amiodarone, early cardioversion).
- ■ Ensure adequate sedative or opioid premedication
  - ➤ Suppress catecholamines, avoid tachyarrhythmias.
  - ➤ But increased risk of respiratory depression (low cardiac output)
- ■ Use fluids & vasoconstrictor agents to treat hypotension
  - ➤ Maintain preload, diastolic perfusion pressure.
  - ➤ Avoid ephedrine, norepinephrine (mixed agonists, increase contractility, may induce tachycardia).

➤ Use a pure vasoconstrictor (phenylephrine); reflex brady-cardia is also helpful.

■ Invasive hemodynamic monitoring, TEE
  ➤ Moderate to large fluid shifts anticipated
  ➤ Presence of symptoms

ANESTHESIA

■ Regional anesthesia is relatively contraindicated
  ➤ Sympathetic block may induce dangerous hypotension, worsen MVO_2
  ➤ Avoid spinal anesthesia (abrupt onset of block)
  ➤ Careful continuous spinal or epidural anesthesia may be tolerated
  ➤ Adequate fluid load before placement (maintain preload)

■ General anesthesia
  ➤ Take measures to maintain slow heart rate & adequate perfusion pressure.
  ➤ Preoxygenate
  ➤ Adequate fluid load before induction (maintain preload)
  ➤ Treat hypotension w/ phenylephrine.
  ➤ Treat tachycardia w/ esmolol.

■ Avoid pancuronium (tachycardia), ketamine (sympath-omimetic).

■ Choose maintenance regimen that maintains slow heart rate, suppresses sympathetic response
  ➤ Avoid isoflurane (increased heart rate); desflurane (increased sympathetic tone).
  ➤ Consider sympatholytic opioid (fentanyl, sufentanil, remifentanil).

WAKE UP AND EMERGENCE

■ Attempt to suppress catecholamines on emergence
  ➤ Judicious use of sympatholytic opioid (fentanyl, sufen-tanil, remifentanil)
  ➤ Avoid morphine (histamine, catecholamine release).

- Consider dexmedetomidine infusion
  - Sympatholytic, provides analgesia w/out respiratory depression
  - Can be continued through tracheal extubation & beyond
  - Dose carefully: can potentiate beta blockade, delay anesthetic emergence
- Potential complications on emergence
  - Delayed emergence (low cardiac output, increased pharmacodynamic effects)
  - Acute myocardial ischemia, pulmonary congestion, edema

ICU AND PACU
- Control pain & anxiety (avoid tachycardia); see above
- Consider short period of postop mechanical ventilation if AS severe
  - Allows controlled emergence
  - Avoids reversal (ie, need for anticholinergic agents [tachycardia])
  - Facilitates evaluation of cardiac, ventilatory function
  - Careful sedation is essential: dexmedetomidine very useful
- Restart preop meds (beta, calcium blockade) as soon as possible.

BRONCHOSPASTIC DISEASE

HUGH PLAYFORD, MD

SCREENING AND EVALUATION
- Consider impact of the asthma & the mgt therapies.
- History of asthma
  - Duration of asthma & triggers
  - Therapy & compliance

➤ Need for ER visit, hospitalizations, intubation & ventilation

➤ Need for systemic steroids & doses

➤ Exercise tolerance

➤ Patient monitoring of asthma severity (peak flow meters)

- Symptoms
  - ➤ Cough
  - ➤ Upper or lower respiratory tract infection
  - ➤ Exercise tolerance
- Signs
  - ➤ Hyperexpansion of thorax
  - ➤ Degree of respiratory distress
  - ➤ Airway obstruction (prolonged expiratory time, wheeze)
  - ➤ Cough
- Investigations
  - ➤ PFTs & spirometry: before & after bronchodilators
  - ➤ Chest x-ray: rarely useful but may help differentiate other causes of respiratory failure
  - ➤ ABGs: if there are concerns regarding the adequacy of ventilation or oxygenation
  - ➤ Sputum MCS: if there are concerns regarding a lower respiratory tract infection

PREOPERATIVE PREPARATION

- Use care w/ preanesthetic agents that may cause respiratory depression.
- Anticholinergic agents may increase viscosity of secretions (preventing adequate clearance).
- H2 receptor antagonists controversial
  - ➤ H2 receptor mediates bronchodilatation; H-1 receptor mediates bronchoconstriction.
  - ➤ H2 receptor antagonist may prevent bronchodilation AND unmask H1-mediated bronchoconstriction.

- Optimally manage any pre-existing airway obstruction
  - Continue pt's usual therapy for asthma to the time of anesthetic induction.
  - Consider chest physiotherapy, systemic hydration, appropriate antibiotics & optimizing bronchodilator therapy.
- For pts on recent & current systemic steroids, supplemental doses of steroids will be needed to prevent unmasking of adrenal suppression.

OPERATIVE PREPARATION
- Goals
  - Specific to the asthma: Optimize any airway obstruction.
  - Specific to anesthesia: Depress airway reflexes to avoid bronchospasm in response to mechanical stimulation.
- Regional anesthesia may be a consideration.

ANESTHESIA
- Goals
  - Have adequate depth of anesthesia during the periods of airway provocation (intubation, incision, extubation).
- Induction agents (benzodiazepines, barbiturates, propofol, etomidate) have little airway reflex depressant actions.
- Ketamine
  - Prevents increased airway resistance better than thiopentone (via the sympathomimetic effect)
  - Increased secretions may counteract this.
- Inhalational agents
  - Used to ensure adequate depth of anesthesia to suppress airway reflexes
  - BUT halothane sensitizes the myocardium to cardiac dysrhythmic effects of beta-agonists & aminophylline.
  - Enflurane, isoflurane & sevoflurane appear as effective as halothane in reversing induced bronchospasm.

- Lidocaine
  - IV bolus (1.5 mg/kg given about 1 min before intubation) may be used to suppress airway reflexes.
  - IV infusion (1–3 mg/kg/hr) may be used to suppress airway reflexes in the place of volatile anesthesia.
  - Intratracheal lidocaine may provide local anesthesia of the upper airway but may also provoke bronchospasm by the presence of the solution.
- Select neuromuscular blockers to minimize the release of histamine.
  - Atracurium has been associated w/ intraop bronchospasm.
  - Succinylcholine associated w/ histamine release but no evidence of increased airway resistance
- Ventilation
  - Avoid the development of pulmonary hyperinflation (gas trapping) or barotraumas.
  - Slow inspiratory rate w/ long I:E ratio to allow sufficient expiratory time for expiratory airflow to return to zero
  - Minimize (or avoid) PEEP.
  - Humidify & warm the inspired gases.
- Maintain adequate hydration (possibly prevent the development of viscous secretions).

WAKE UP AND EMERGENCE
- Aim to extubate while anesthesia is sufficient to suppress airway hyperresponsiveness.
- Lidocaine (IV bolus or infusion may be useful)

ICU OR PACU
N/A

CARCINOID SYNDROME

GIUDITTA ANGELINI, MD

SCREENING & EVALUATION

N/A

PREOPERATIVE PREPARATION

- In general, preoperative course reflects intraoperative course.

OPERATIVE PREPARATION

N/A

ANESTHESIA

- Variable depending on degree of hormone secretion
- 50% of pts w/ intraoperative bronchospasm may have no previous history.
- Benzodiazepine premedication
  - Anxiety can trigger carcinoid episode.
- 100 mcg octreotide given on induction
- Smooth induction w/ propofol or etomidate & nondepolarizer
  - Hypotension, hypertension, hypercapnia can trigger carcinoid episode.
  - Thiopental & succinylcholine can release histamine.
- Use fentanyl & derivatives.
  - Morphine can release histamine.
- Arterial line for BP monitoring
- Central line may be indicated for fluid resuscitation w/ or w/out pulmonary artery catheter for pts w/ cardiac disease.
- General or regional anesthesia acceptable
- Direct & indirect sympathomimetic drugs can stimulate release of hormones, so treat hypotension w/ octreotide & fluid.

- Treat hypertension w/ octreotide & increased anesthesia.
- Treat bronchospasm w/ octreotide & inhaled ipratropium.

WAKE UP & EMERGENCE
N/A

ICU OR PACU
- Monitor blood glucose closely.

CHEMOTHERAPEUTIC AGENTS

JONATHAN T. KETZLER, MD

SCREENING AND EVALUATION
- Anthracyclines
  - There are no tests to determine which pts will develop heart failure.
  - Do gated radionucleotide blood pooled study or echocardiogram as baseline before patient receives a cumulative dose of 400 mg/m^2 & before each following treatment.
  - Because injury can continue for years after treatment, ideally a full cardiac evaluation should be done within 1 month of elective surgery.
- Bleomycin
  - Chest x-ray & pulmonary function tests to evaluate for pneumonitis & pulmonary fibrosis

PREOP PREPARATION
OPERATIVE PREPARATION
N/A

ANESTHESIA
- Anthracyclines
  - Avoid cardiodepressant drugs.

> May need pulmonary artery catheter or intraoperative transesophageal echocardiography if cardiac function is in question
- Bleomycin
  > Avoid supplemental oxygen; keep as close to FIO_2 of 0.21 as oxygenation permits.
  > If pulmonary compliance is low, alternative modes of ventilation may be needed. Consider ICU ventilator & total IV anesthesia

WAKE UP & EMERGENCE

N/A

ICU OR PACU
- See recommendations under "Anesthesia."

CHRONIC OBSTRUCTIVE PULMONARY DISEASE (COPD)

HUGH R. PLAYFORD, MBBS

SCREENING & EVALUATION
- Assess for severity of disease & any reversible components (reactive airway disease, infection).
- Aside from history & examination, consider PFTs, ABGs, sputum culture & sensitivity.
- GOLD Guidelines: classification of severity of COPD

Stage	Classification
0: At risk	Normal spirometry
	Chronic symptoms (cough, sputum production)
1: Mild COPD	FEV1/FVC <70%
	FEV1 >80% predicted
	W/ or w/out chronic symptoms (cough, sputum production)

2: Moderate COPD	FEV1/FVC <70% 30% > FEV1 <80% predicted W/ or w/out chronic symptoms (cough, sputum production, dyspnea)
3: Severe COPD	FEV1/FVC <70% FEV1 <30% predicted or FEV1 <50% predicted plus respiratory failure or clinical signs of right heart failure

- Identify & eradicate acute bacterial infection w/ antibiotics & physical therapy.
- Optimize the strength of skeletal muscles (nutrition, physical therapy, avoidance of hypokalemia).
- Smoking
  - ➤ Smoking associated w/ increased postop pulmonary complications
  - ➤ Carbon monoxide leads to increased carboxyhemoglobin, tissue hypoxia, shift of oxygen dissociation curve; elimination half-time for carbon monoxide about 4–6 hrs.
  - ➤ Smoking also induces mucus hypersecretion, impairment of mucociliary transport & small airway narrowing; these recover slowly after smoking cessation (up to 8 wks).
  - ➤ Immune system interference (need about 6 wks of cessation to recover)
  - ➤ Hepatic enzyme recovery after 6–8 wks of abstinence
  - ➤ But smokers have lower incidence of DVT after surgery.
  - ➤ Recommend that pt cease smoking before elective surgery.

PREOPERATIVE PREPARATION
- Eradicate any pulmonary infection.
- Optimize pulmonary therapy.
- Consider physical therapy & nutrition.
- Pts are at increased risk of developing acute respiratory failure during postop period.

- Plan intraoperative technique (regional, general, combined) & postop analgesic regimen to have minimal pulmonary detriment.
- Postop impairment of pulmonary function likely w/:
  - Any chronic disease that involves the lung
  - Smoking history, persistent cough, and/or wheezing
  - Chest wall & spinal deformities
  - Morbid obesity
  - Requirement for single lung anesthesia or lung resection
  - Neuromuscular disease

OPERATIVE PREPARATION
- Bronchodilators rarely improve the FEV1 by >10%.
- Anticholinergic therapy
- Antibiotics
- Influenza vaccination
- Diuresis for cor pulmonale & right heart failure
- Supplemental oxygen titrated to the individual pt's needs
- Physical training programs

ANESTHESIA
- Regional anesthesia
  - Potentially avoids respiratory depressant effects of sedative drugs
  - Avoid regional techniques that provide sensory anesthesia above T6 (may decrease expiratory reserve volume & impair effectiveness to cough & clear secretions)
- General anesthesia
  - Use care w/ COPD pts w/ some airway reactivity: these pts may develop significant laryngospasm and/or bronchospasm w/ airway instrumentation.
  - Volatile anesthesia allows humidification, anesthesia delivery w/ a relatively rapid onset & offset, blunting of airway reflexes & reflex bronchospasm & volatile-induced bronchodilatation.

➤ Volatile anesthesia also attenuates regional hypoxic pulmonary vasoconstriction, leading to increased R-to-L intrapulmonary shunting.

➤ Avoid nitrous oxide in the presence of pulmonary bullae (nitrous oxide leads to enlargement & rupture & possible tension pneumothorax).

➤ Nitrous oxide technique also limits the FiO_2 that can be delivered.

➤ Opioids may lead to prolonged respiratory depression; use judiciously.

➤ Humidification is used to prevent drying of secretions in the airways.

➤ Ventilation
  • Principles are to allow adequate minute ventilation & adequate minute ventilation & minimize the risk of barotrauma & dynamic pulmonary hyperinflation (which can impair ventilation & circulation).
  • Tidal volume around 10 mL/kg, slow respiratory rate around 6–10 breaths/min
  • Slow respiratory rate allows a long expiratory time to reduce the risk of dynamic pulmonary hyperinflation.
  • May need to follow ABGs in addition to continuous pulse oximetry & capnography.

WAKE UP & EMERGENCE

■ Principles are to have the pt well analgesed w/ good effective cough & deep inspiration w/out any residual respiratory depression.

■ Extubation
  ➤ Ideally, extubate at the end of the surgical procedure (depends on procedure & duration of anesthesia).
  ➤ Tracheal tube increases airway resistance & risk of reflex bronchoconstriction, limits the pt's ability to clear secretions effectively & increases the risk of iatrogenic infection.

- Analgesia
  - Regional techniques using local anesthesia and/or neuraxial opioids may be able to avoid significant respiratory depression.
  - Neuraxial local anesthesia may lead to postural hypotension & interfere w/ postop ambulation & sputum clearance & incentive spirometry.
  - Pt-controlled analgesia w/ systemic opioids may also minimize the risk of significant respiratory depression.
  - With any route of opioid, however, potent respiratory depression may develop; epidural opioids may depress ventilation up to 12 hrs after administration.
  - Consider other nonrespiratory-depressing analgesics as adjunctive agents (acetaminophen, alpha-2 agonists such as clonidine & dexmedetomidine, NSAIDs).
- Chest physical therapy & incentive spirometry

ICU OR PACU
- Continued intubation & ventilation in the postop period may be necessary in pts w/ severe COPD and/or major upper abdominal or thoracic surgery.
- Discontinuation of ventilation is based on the pt's clinical condition (preexisting pulmonary impairment, surgical procedure, duration of anesthesia) as well as indices of respiratory function.
  - The changes in pulmonary function that occur postop are primarily restrictive; these changes added to preexisting COPD may be catastrophic in the individual pt.
  - Proportional decreases in all lung volumes, no change in airway resistance
  - FRC decreases from decreased abdominal excursion (eg, from abdominal operations), abnormal postop respiratory pattern (shallow, rapid breaths).

➤ Operative site is the most important factor: non-laparoscopic upper abdominal operations decrease FRC by 40–50% > lower abdominal & thoracic decrease FRC by 30% > other operative sites decrease FRC by 15–20%.

CHRONIC RENAL FAILURE

ROBERT N. SLADEN, MD

SCREENING AND EVALUATION

■ Note the following:
  ➤ Etiology of chronic renal failure (ie, presence of systemic disease)
  ➤ Urine output (oliguric or polyuric)
  ➤ Type of dialysis (HD or CAPD) & most recent treatment
  ➤ Treatment w/ human recombinant erythropoietin (EPO)
■ Look for physical signs of anemia, LVH, CHF, neuropathy, sepsis, malnutrition. Examine shunt sites and/or CAPD catheter site for infection.
■ Relevant lab studies
  ➤ Hct (anemia), CBC (leukocytosis)
  ➤ Electrolytes (assess acidosis by total CO2 if ABG impracticable)
  ➤ BUN, creatinine (look for recent change)
  ➤ Ivy bleeding time (BT) (>15 min: platelet dysfunction)
  ➤ ECG (LVH, hyperkalemia)
  ➤ Chest x-ray (LVH, pulmonary congestion or edema)

PREOPERATIVE PREPARATION

■ Hemodialysis
  ➤ Schedule day before elective surgery to avoid acute fluid & electrolyte shifts.

- CAPD
  - ➤ Continue until time of surgery.
  - ➤ Assess excessive abdominal girth (may compromise functional residual capacity).
- Preop blood transfusion only for:
  - ➤ Acute blood loss
  - ➤ Cardiopulmonary disease
  - ➤ Major surgery with Hct <28%
- Transfuse during dialysis only:
  - ➤ Avoid fluid overload & hyperkalemia.
- Correct platelet dysfunction before major surgery:
  - ➤ DDAVP 0.3 micrograms/kg over 20 min, or
  - ➤ Cryoprecipitate 10 units (preferred if exposure to catecholamines)
- Control labile/symptomatic hypertension
- Preop alpha-2 agonists (clonidine or guanabenz)
  - ➤ Clonidine transdermal patch to prevent rebound hypertension

OPERATIVE PREPARATION
- Minimize sedative or opioid premeds.
- Aspiration prophylaxis
  - ➤ Anticholinergic agent (glycopyrrolate preferred)
  - ➤ H_2 blocker (famotidine preferred: least likelihood of thrombocytopenia)
  - ➤ Metoclopramide
  - ➤ Sodium bicitrate
- Use universal & aseptic precautions throughout
  - ➤ Avoid BP cuffs or arterial catheters on arm w/ AV fistula/shunt.
  - ➤ Avoid urinary catheter in anuric or oliguric pts.
- Invasive hemodynamic monitoring
  - ➤ If large fluid shifts anticipated
  - ➤ Sepsis

➤ Cardiopulmonary insufficiency
■ Avoid pressure or stretch on fistula sites, bony prominences, joints
➤ Sensory neuropathy (pts do not feel positional discomfort)
➤ Renal osteodystrophy (fragile bones & joints)
■ Use active warming devices to prevent hypothermia
➤ Forced-air convection blanket
■ Consider intraoperative hemodialysis during CPB.

ANESTHESIA
■ Regional anesthesia
➤ Not contraindicated if coagulopathy corrected
➤ Avoid if increased risk of hypotension (autonomic neuropathy), infection.
➤ Watch for postop pulmonary edema (sympathetic block wears off, increase in SVR).
■ General anesthesia
➤ Aspiration precautions (head up, rapid sequence, cricoid pressure)
➤ Preoxygenate
➤ Adequate fluid load (250–1,000 mL) prior to induction
■ Succinylcholine is not contraindicated if:
➤ Serum K <5.0 mEq/L
➤ Pt dialyzed within last 24 hrs
■ Avoid pancuronium & pipecuronium (prolonged action).
■ After tracheal intubation, increase minute ventilation
➤ Compensate for chronic metabolic acidosis
■ Keep maintenance fluids to a minimum but fully replace fluid losses.
■ Enflurane (fluoride), sevoflurane (compound A)
➤ Theoretical possibility of nephrotoxicity
■ Anticipate labile BP
➤ Hypotension (deep anesthesia, fluid losses, positional changes)

- ➤ Hypertension (inadequate anesthesia)
- ➤ Beta blockers or calcium blockers are helpful for control.
- ■ Anticipate hyperkalemia
  - ➤ Evoked by high-dose beta blockade
  - ➤ Protects against digoxin-induced arrhythmias but may exacerbate conduction block

WAKE UP AND EMERGENCE
- ■ Anesthetic emergence may be delayed
  - ➤ Pharmacokinetic (delayed elimination, active metabolites)
  - ➤ Pharmacodynamic (enhanced sensitivity to effects)
- ■ Potential complications on emergence
  - ➤ Vomiting, aspiration
  - ➤ Hypertension
  - ➤ Persistent neuromuscular blockade
  - ➤ Respiratory depression
  - ➤ Pulmonary edema

ICU OR PACU
- ■ Chronic metabolic acidosis + CO_2 retention: acute acidosis, hyperkalemia
- ■ Consider short period of postop mechanical ventilation
  - ➤ Allows controlled emergence
  - ➤ Avoids reversal agents
  - ➤ Facilitates evaluation of neurologic, ventilatory function
- ■ Restrict maintenance fluid; replace sequestration or overt losses.
- ■ Anticipate & treat hyperkalemia.
- ■ Hemodialysis
  - ➤ Severe uremia, hyperkalemia, acidosis, acute fluid overload
  - ➤ Risk of hemodynamic instability, myocardial ischemia
- ■ Peritoneal dialysis
  - ➤ Hemodynamically stable

- ➤ Slow; not suited for severe uremia, hyperkalemia, acidosis, acute fluid overload
- ➤ Abdominal distention may compromise functional residual capacity.
- ■ Continuous venovenous hemofiltration/dialysis (CVVH/D)
  - ➤ Large-volume removal w/ stable hemodynamics
  - ➤ Requires heparin, may promote bleeding

COCAINE TOXICITY

MARY E. McSWEENEY, MD

SCREENING AND EVALUATION

- ■ History: most pts deny drug abuse; often associated w/ alcohol, tobacco & other illicit drug use
- ■ Physical exam: tachycardia, angina, tachypnea, agitation
- ■ Metabolites: urine positive for cocaine metabolites (benzoylecgonine, ecgonine methyl ester) for 72 hrs. Cocaine & ethanol used in combination is extremely common; look for metabolite (cocaethylene).

PREOPERATIVE PREPARATION

- ■ Hypertension: use nitroglycerin, labetalol, phentolamine & hydralazine for control; conventional wisdom is to avoid propranolol (beta blockade) because of potential for unopposed alpha-adrenergic stimulation, which exacerbates cocaine-induced vasoconstriction
- ■ Hypotension: likely ephedrine-resistant; use phenylephrine (alpha agonist)
- ■ Tachycardia: use combined alpha/beta antagonist (labetalol)
- ■ Agitation & acute coronary syndrome associated w/ cocaine toxicity: first-line treatment nitrates, benzodiazepines & oxygen (aspirin if not contraindicated before surgery), then as indicated above

OPERATIVE PREPARATION

- Monitoring
  - ➤ V5 lead ECG, temperature, pulse oximetry, $ETCO_2$
  - ➤ Consider arterial line, central line, urine catheter & PA catheter if myocardial ischemia or dysfunction suspected.

ANESTHESIA

- Anesthetic
  - ➤ Halothane may be avoided due to sensitization of myocardium to catecholamines.
  - ➤ Regional anesthesia can be used.
- Controlling hypertension & tachycardia
  - ➤ Nitroglycerine 0.5–2.0 mcg/kg/min IV
  - ➤ Phentolamine 1–5 mg IV q5min or 1 mg/min continuous infusion
  - ➤ Labetalol 10–20 mg IV q10min to maximum 200 mg
  - ➤ Esmolol 10–20 mg IV q10min or 50–300 mcg/kg/min continuous
  - ➤ Hydralazine 10 mg IV q30min to maximum 40 mg
- Treating arrhythmias
  - ➤ Lidocaine okay for treatment of VF & VT
  - ➤ Consider $NaHCO_3$ in presence of acidosis; decreases QRS prolongation & incidence of VT
  - ➤ Avoid epinephrine.
  - ➤ Avoid IA antiarrhythmics (quinidine, procainamide, disopyramide); they exacerbate prolongation of QRS & QT.

WAKE UP & EMERGENCE

N/A

ICU OR PACU

- ICU care for pts w/ cocaine toxicity

■ Altered pain perception (due to abnormalities in endorphin levels & changes in mu & kappa opioid receptor densities) makes postop pain mgt a challenge in this population.

CONGESTIVE HEART FAILURE

MUHAMMED ITANI, MD, AND JONATHAN T. KETZLER, MD

SCREENING AND EVALUATION

■ Symptoms of left & right ventricular failure (LVF, RVF)
  ➤ Fatigue, dyspnea at rest, orthopnea, ankle swelling, loss of appetite
■ History & physical exam
  ➤ Tachypnea, crackles: pulmonary congestion/edema (LVF)
  ➤ S4, S3 heart sound (LVF)
■ Peripheral edema & JVD (LVF, RVF)
■ Chest x-ray
  ➤ Cardiomegaly, pulmonary congestion, edema & pleural effusion
  ➤ Early signs of LV: pulmonary venous distention, perivascular edema
  ➤ Kerley lines (septal edema): A (upper), B (lower), C (base w/ honeycomb pattern)
  ➤ Late signs: interstitial & alveolar edema, pleural & subpleural effusions
  ➤ Chest x-ray may lag behind worsening (up to 12 hrs) & improving (up to 4 days) CHF
■ EKG
  ➤ Cardiomyopathy: poor R-wave progression
  ➤ Prolonged conduction, LBBB, RBBB.
  ➤ Varying degrees of conduction disease (first-, second- or third-degree HB)
  ➤ Evidence of old MI

PREOPERATIVE PREPARATION

- Chronic therapy goal is to slow LV remodeling & dilated cardiomyopathy.
  - ➤ Dietary control: low-sodium diet
  - ➤ Regular exercise
  - ➤ Diuretics: decrease pulmonary congestion w/out excessive hypovolemia
  - ➤ Long-term nitrates
- Acute treatment to relieve congestion & improve tissue perfusion
  - ➤ Restoration & maintenance of sinus rhythm (pharmacologic, cardioversion)
  - ➤ Diuretics: decrease pulmonary congestion w/out excessive decrease in preload
  - ➤ Correction of precipitating factor (ischemia, hypertension)
  - ➤ Inodilators (inotropic support + afterload reduction)
    - Catecholamines: dobutamine
    - Phosphodiesterase inhibitors: milrinone
- Invasive options
  - ➤ Angioplasty or CABG to relieve CHF due to CAD
  - ➤ Surgical valve repair to relieve valve problems
  - ➤ Intra-aortic balloon counterpulsation (bridge to emergency surgery)
  - ➤ Heart transplant
  - ➤ Ventricular assist devices (VAD): useful to unload the heart & help recover its function; used mainly as bridge to heart transplant
  - ➤ Acute treatment to relieve congestion & improve tissue perfusion

OPERATIVE PREPARATION

- Delay surgery if cardiac status is not optimized.
- Administer oxygen preop to avoid hypoxia.

- Avoid dehydration and/or fluid overload.
- For major surgery, consider invasive hemodynamic monitoring:
  - ➤ Arterial line, CVP (access for vasoactive drugs)
  - ➤ PA catheter
  - ➤ Intraop TEE

ANESTHESIA
- Induction: ketamine is useful
  - ➤ Sympathomimetics may preserve BP: ketamine, desflurane
  - ➤ Avoid potent cardiac depressant agents: thiopental, propofol, nitrous oxide.
  - ➤ Judicious dosing of etomidate, opioids & benzodiazepines
  - ➤ Use volatile anesthetic agents w/ caution due to cardiodepressant effect.
- Maintenance
  - ➤ May use opioids as the sole maintenance agents
  - ➤ Choice of neuromuscular blocking agent (NMBA): avoid histamine releasers
  - ➤ Positive-pressure ventilation may decrease pulmonary congestion & improve oxygenation.
  - ➤ Inotropic drugs (dobutamine, milrinone) may be needed intraoperatively to optimize cardiac function.
  - ➤ Regional anesthesia can be used safely & may improve cardiac output & decrease PVR.
  - ➤ Spinal & rapid epidural anesthesia may precipitate severe hypotension.

WAKE UP & EMERGENCE
- Do not extubate until hemodynamically stable & pulmonary edema under control.

➤ Residual anesthesia may compromise ability to provide work of breathing required for pulmonary congestion/edema.

➤ Removal of positive pressure can precipitate acute pulmonary edema.

➤ Upper airway obstruction will exacerbate pulmonary congestion/edema (negative pressure edema).

ICU OR PACU

■ Consider a period of postop mechanical ventilation (see Wake Up & Emergence).

■ Rule out MI.
  ➤ New Q waves on ECG
  ➤ Troponin > 2 ng/mL > 8 hrs after non-cardiac surgery

■ Aggressive pain control to avoid sympathetic activation & worsening of pulmonary edema

■ Avoid/anticipate abrupt cessation of spinal or epidural anesthesia:
  ➤ Abrupt cessation of sympathetic block
  ➤ Abrupt increase in afterload
  ➤ May provoke acute CHF/pulmonary edema

■ Continue & adjust inotropic support & preload/afterload reduction.

COR PULMONALE AND RHF

MUHAMMED ITANI, MD, AND JONATHAN T. KETZLER, MD

SCREENING AND EVALUATION

■ Evaluate etiology of cor pulmonale & severity of pulmonary pathology (see "Diseases" section).

■ PFTs, ABGs (evaluate severity of COPD)

■ Chest x-ray

> Decreased retrosternal space on lateral view (RVH)
> Prominent main PA
> Decreased pulmonary vascular markings (pulmonary hypertension)
> Heart size may change between acute episodes.

■ EKG
> Peaked P wave in leads II, III & AVF
> Right axis deviation & complete or incomplete RBBB
> CBC, electrolytes: secondary polycythemia, leukocytosis (active infection), K (digoxin therapy)

■ TTE
> Assess RV function, RV systolic pressure.
> RA size, tricuspid valve

■ Right heart cath
> PA pressure, RVEDP, RV function
> Trial of IV or inhaled pulmonary vasodilators (nitric oxide, prostacyclin)
> If response (80% of PPH): use in OR.

PREOPERATIVE PREPARATION

■ Anticipate physiologic & pharmacologic factors that increase PVR:
> Arterial hypoxemia
> Hypercarbia
> Acidosis
> High doses of vasoconstrictor catecholamines (epinephrine, norepinephrine)

■ Judicious diuresis to relieve RV overload (RV is preload dependent)

■ Digoxin: increased risk of digitoxicity
> Exacerbated by hypoxemia, acidosis & hypokalemia

■ Calcium channel blockers: effective in 33% of pts

■ Treat active infection (commonly *Haemophilus, Pneumococcus*)

- Anticoagulation: transition pts on coumadin for AF to IV heparin.
- Pts on IV prostacyclin
- Anticipate platelet inhibition & bleeding.
- Anticipate hypotension & arterial hypoxemia.

OPERATIVE PREPARATION
- Avoid heavy premedication.
  - Sedatives, opioids suppress ventilatory drive.
  - Psychological support may be more effective!
- Avoid anticholinergic agents (decrease the ability to clear secretions).
- Maintain hydration (RV preload).
- Obtain baseline ABGs.

ANESTHESIA
- Induction
  - Preoxygenation
  - Ensure adequate fluid loading prior to induction:
    - Acute vasodilation is poorly tolerated.
    - RV unable to generate increased flow because of high PVR
    - LV preload inadequate
    - Profound refractory systemic hypotension may result.
    - Low systemic pressure + high PA pressure: risk of RV ischemia
  - Judicious IV induction (decrease doses 50–60%)
  - Ensure adequate anesthetic depth for endotracheal intubation:
    - Avoid bronchospasm, pulmonary vasoconstriction.
- Maintenance & monitoring
- Consider arterial line & CVP
- Frequent ABGs
- Assess RV preload & response to PVR

- Access for vasoactive drugs
  - Consider PA catheter for major surgery, large fluid shifts
  - Maintenance
    - TIVA (titrate dosage to avoid postop ventilatory depression)
    - Low-dose volatile agents (avoid myocardial depression)
    - Avoid rapid increase in desflurane concentration: increased PVR.
    - Avoid N_2O w/ TIVA: increases PVR.
  - Judicious hyperventilation
    - Mild respiratory alkalosis protects against increase in PVR.
  - Regional anesthesia
    - Sympathetic blockade poorly tolerated in pts w/ high PVR (hypotension)
    - Avoid spinal anesthesia; careful titration of epidural block.

WAKE UP & EMERGENCE

- Anticipate & treat physiologic & pharmacologic factors that increase PVR:
  - Arterial hypoxemia
  - Hypercarbia
  - Acidosis
  - Pain (increased endogenous catecholamines)
- Wake up
  - In selected cases, consider extubation under deep anesthesia.
    - Avoid bronchoconstriction, increased PVR.
  - Judicious titration of fentanyl and/or dexmedetomidine
    - Goal is smooth emergence w/out pain.

ICU OR PACU

- Anticipate & treat physiologic & pharmacologic factors that increase PVR:

- ➤ Arterial hypoxemia
- ➤ Hypercarbia
- ➤ Acidosis
- ➤ Pain (increased endogenous catecholamines)
- ➤ Exogenous vasoconstrictor catecholamines (epinephrine, norepinephrine)
- ➤ Arginine vasopressin (AVP 1–4 u/hr) useful in vasodilated shock
  - • Increases SVR ≫ than PVR
- ■ Avoid excess opioids & sedatives that provoke hypercarbia.
- ■ Hemodynamic mgt as above (ensure adequate RV preload, decrease PVR)
- ■ Severe, labile pulmonary hypertension
  - ➤ Inhaled nitric oxide (selective, expensive)
  - ➤ Inhaled prostacyclin (less selective, inexpensive)

DIABETES MELLITUS AND DIABETIC EMERGENCIES

DOUGLAS B. COURSIN, MD

SCREENING AND EVALUATION

- ■ Diabetics have surgery & procedures more commonly than non-diabetics.
- ■ 1/3 to 1/2 of pts w/ diabetes do not know it at the time of surgery.
- ■ Risk for perioperative complications greater for diabetics
- ■ Tighter control limits long-term microvascular disease.
- ■ History
  - ➤ Does pt measure sugars? What do they run?
  - ➤ How does pt respond to insulin?
  - ➤ Does pt know what it feels like to have a hypoglycemic reaction? How does pt treat it?
  - ➤ Signs or symptoms of autonomic or peripheral neuropathy, ischemic hart disease, CHF, renal insufficiency

- Physical exam
  - Loss of beat-to-beat variability in pulse, orthostasis, stocking/glove sensory loss
  - Rales, peripheral edema, S4 (hypertension), S3 (CHF)
- Type 1 absolute insulin deficiency
  - Always need a basal amount of insulin or will convert to ketogenesis
  - At risk for DKA
  - Frequently have micro- & macrovascular disease involving the eye, peripheral vasculature, heart, kidneys, peripheral & autonomic nervous system
    - Should screen for this in history, physical & individualized lab evaluation
- Type 2 DM develops secondary to relative deficiency of insulin or insulin hyporesponsiveness or resistance
  - May or may not require oral hypoglycemics and/or insulin
  - Many pts are obese & inactive, but increasing recognition of younger (<25–30 yrs) active pts w/ a genetic predisposition to type 2
  - Tighter control chronically may be beneficial.
  - Improved control perioperatively should be the goal to limit infections & exacerbation of ischemia.
- Routine screening tests as needed
  - Fasting blood sugar
  - Urinalysis: check for albuminuria, WBCs, bacteria
  - BUN/creatinine
  - ECG: if history, signs or symptoms of ischemia, age > 40, undergoing major vascular or cardiac surgery

PREOPERATIVE PREPARATION
- Identify end-organ compromise.
- Optimize end-organ function & take steps to limit end-organ insult
  - Heart

- If diastolic dysfunction, aim to keep heart rate slow & to use agents that optimize diastolic relaxation
- Beta block when needed & as able
- CHF increasingly common w/ age; diuretics may be associated with various electrolyte abnormalities, hypokalemia, hyponatremia, hypomagnesemia
- Ischemia may be silent.
- Recommend ECG if >40 yrs or earlier if suspected or known ischemia/infarct. Compare as able to older ECG.

➤ Kidney
- Adequate hydration & intravascular fluid maintenance
- N-acetyl cysteine (NAC) if creatinine >1.5–1.8 mg/dL & contrast used

OPERATIVE PREPARATION
- ■ Premedication
  - ➤ Individualize
  - ➤ Use of antacids, metoclopramide, H2 blocker, and/or proton pump inhibitor as needed

ANESTHESIA
- ■ Technique
  - ➤ General, regional or local as indicated
  - ➤ Document neurologic status, coagulation function & site suitability prior to initiation of a neuraxial or major regional block.
  - ➤ Some advocate general over regional in pts w/ significant baseline neuropathy, uncontrollable airway or regional site compromise.
  - ➤ Amputations for advanced peripheral vascular disease may be augmented by concurrent advanced peripheral neuropathy.
- ■ Induction
  - ➤ Increased risk for aspiration
  - ➤ Increased risk of difficult intubation

- Particularly type 1 diabetics: 40% reported as difficult
- Look for stiff joint syndrome
  - Positive prayer sign when approximate palms of the hands
  - Immobility of head & neck & other joints
- Consider awake, fiberoptic intubation; plan for difficult airway management: see algorithm
- ➤ Presence of hyperglycemia & volume depletion and/or autonomic neuropathy may make pts more susceptible to hypotension secondary to induction agents such as thiopental & propofol.
  - Consider etomidate if cardiovascular or volume compromise.
  - Consider adjusted dose to avoid bolus effect.
- ➤ Positioning is crucial; higher incidence of skin & nerve injury
  - Careful padding; avoid extension, compression injury, burns
- ■ Maintenance
  - ➤ Total IV anesthesia
  - ➤ Inhaled
    - Choice based on speed onset/offset, metabolism, renal function, cost
  - ➤ Type 1 diabetics or those w/ coronary artery disease, bowel obstruction or other contraindication, avoid N_2O to limit altered homocysteine & methionine metabolism abnormalities, gas expansion

WAKE UP AND EMERGENCE

- ■ Risk for aspiration
- ■ Risk of sympathetic response in pts w/ suspected or known ischemia
- ■ If slow to awaken, obtain stat glucose to rule hypoglycemia.

ICU OR PACU

- ■ Measure blood glucose at arrival to PACU/ICU.

- Increased risk for aspiration because of gastroparesis
- Diabetics require postop critical care more than non-diabetics.
- Increasing evidence that euglycemia (80–110 mg/dL) is the goal for critically ill pts.
  - Use of insulin and/or insulin/glucose/potassium infusions advocated
    - Use regular insulin as infusion
    - Reliable insulin absorption if IV
    - Careful follow-up of blood glucose, potassium levels. Prone to hypoglycemia, esp. if reversing DKA & when drive glucose & potassium into the cell.
- Greater incidence of ischemia & worse outcome neurologically & cardiovascularly if ischemia develops
  - Can improve this by maintaining euglycemia
  - Postop MI
  - Postop stroke
  - Postop infection
  - Postop neuropathy
- Diabetic emergencies: hypoglycemia, DKA, nonketotic hyperosmolar state (NKHS)
- Hypoglycemia
  - More common in type 1 than type 2
  - Increased incidence in pts on ACE inhibitors
  - Crucial to avoid prolonged hypoglycemia
  - Symptoms are neuroglycopenic
    - Confusion, altered mental status, agitation progressing to somnolence, coma & eventually death
  - Treat w/ IV glucose
    - Bolus 1/2 to 1 amp of D50, then follow w/ an infusion of D5 to D10W & serial blood glucose measurements
- DKA & NKHS are related states
  - DKA mainly in type 1, NKHS usually in older type 2
  - Both have significant hyperglycemia & hyperosmolarity. Significant osmotic diuresis; as they progress, pt

becomes acidotic, develops multiple electrolyte abnormalities & may become increasingly depressed neurologically. These are medical emergencies requiring aggressive, timely intervention. Significant morbidity & mortality, usually from precipitating event.

■ DKA: mainly type 1 but may occur in type 2 pts who chronically receive insulin

➤ Usually precipitated by infection (most commonly respiratory or urinary tract) or stress
  • May be precipitated by:
    • Trauma, surgery/critical illness (MI, stroke, pancreatitis)
    • Failure to take insulin
    • Alcohol, drug use
    • Corticosteroid use or large doses of thiazide diuretics
    • Overexertion, heat stroke, inadequate oral intake, esp. in elderly

➤ Blood glucose usually <800–900 mg/dL
  • Hyperglycemia results in severe polyuria & polydipsia.

➤ Volume-depleted, acidotic, multiple electrolyte abnormalities
  • Need fluid resuscitation
    • Usually 3–6 L depleted
    • Initial replacement is w/ normal saline, then change to 1/2 normal saline to aid replacement of free water deficit & avoid hypernatremia
    • May add 20–40 mEq KCl to each liter of 1/2 normal saline to replete K+ deficits (if pt has reasonable renal function & is making urine). This is equivalent of 3/4 normal saline.
  • IV insulin, bolus 5–20 units, then infusion at 5–10 units an hour. Aim to lower blood glucose by 100 mg/dL per hour; start dextrose infusion when blood glucose is around 250 mg/dL.

- Maintain insulin infusion until serum ketones are completely cleared.
- Correct electrolyte abnormalities
  - May be hyponatremic, but often spurious; as replace fluids, change to 1/2 normal saline to replace free water deficit & avoid hypernatremia
  - May develop severe hypokalemia as volume replete & acidosis clears
  - May need large amounts of potassium
    - Osmotic diuresis losses of K+
    - K+/H+ cellular shifts as acidosis corrected
  - May need magnesium & phosphorus replacement
    - May use K_2PO_4 as part of replacement for hypokalemia
  - Rarely need HCO_3; if used, watch for overcorrection & metabolic alkalosis
- Cerebral edema a major complication, esp. for children
  - Care w/ overcorrecting of glucose
- NKHS
  - Older pts, more commonly type 2
  - Little accumulation of ketoacids
  - Blood glucose frequently >1,000 mg/dL
  - Severe volume resuscitation: 8–10 L deficits
    - Initial resuscitation w/ normal saline. since pt is salt & water depleted
  - May be very sensitive to insulin, so watch glucose carefully

---

EPILEPSY

GEBHARD WAGENER, MD

SCREENING AND EVALUATION
- Causes for seizures:
  - Hyponatremia

- ➤ Hypoglycemia
- ➤ Other electrolyte abnormalities
- ➤ Drug intoxication
- ➤ Intracranial hemorrhage
- ➤ Increased ICP
- ➤ Cyclosporin-induced seizures
- ➤ ETOH withdrawal
- ■ Surgical treatment of seizure disorder
  - ➤ For severe treatment-resistant seizure disorder
  - ➤ 1/3 have no seizures after surgery, 1/3 less frequent seizures, 1/3 no change.
    - • Morbidity (hemiparesis & other neurologic deficits): 1–3%
- ■ History/exam
  - ➤ Nature, cause & frequency of seizures
  - ➤ Date of last seizure
  - ➤ Meds: last change of medication or dose
  - ➤ Focused neurologic exam: rule out:
    - • Peripheral neuropathies
    - • Increased ICP
  - ➤ Surgical treatment of seizure disorder
    - • Location of seizure focus
- ■ Investigations
  - ➤ Antiepileptic drug levels
  - ➤ CBC
  - ➤ LFT: drug-induced hepatic dysfunction
  - ➤ Coagulation profile: valproic acid
  - ➤ Consider MRI, CT if increased ICP suspected.
  - ➤ Surgical treatment of seizure disorder
    - • MRI, CT, cortical mapping, functional MRI, PET scan, water test to detect right/left hemispheric dominance

PREOPERATIVE PREPARATION
- ■ Antiepileptic agents to be taken on day of surgery
- ■ Surgical treatment of seizure disorder

➤ Pt will likely be off seizure meds to elicit seizure focus.

OPERATIVE PREPARATION

■ Surgical treatment of seizure disorder
  ➤ Mostly awake craniotomy: inform pt about need for cooperation, possibility of intraop awareness
  ➤ With head frame in place, no access to airway; fiberoptic scope for intubation should be available in case of neurologic complications (stroke, hemorrhage)

ANESTHESIA

■ Barbiturates, benzodiazepine, inhalational agents & propofol increase seizure threshold (historical: enflurane decreases seizure threshold).
■ Propofol-induced opisthotonos is not seizure-related.
■ Etomidate induces myoclonus but does not decrease seizure threshold.
■ Avoid ketamine.
■ Avoid methohexital; can activate epileptogenic foci.
■ Surgical treatment of seizure disorder
  ➤ Low-dose benzodiazepines, propofol for awake craniotomy. Benzodiazepines can be antagonized with flumazenil.
  ➤ Methohexital may be used to provoke seizures.

WAKE UP AND EMERGENCE

■ Avoid hypercarbia & hyper-/hypotension in case of increased ICP.
■ Emergence may be delayed: enzyme induction
■ Surgical treatment of seizure disorder
  ➤ New neurologic deficits require immediate intervention: CT scan & possible re-exploration for hemorrhage.

ICU OR PACU

■ Depends on extent of surgery & condition of pt
■ Surgical treatment of seizure disorder
  ➤ Observe pt in neurological intensive care unit.

THE GERIATRIC PATIENT

HUGH R. PLAYFORD, MD

SCREENING AND EVALUATION
- Need to consider:
  - Effects of aging per se
  - Comorbidities
  - Pharmacotherapy

PREOPERATIVE PREPARATION
N/A

OPERATIVE PREPARATION
N/A

ANESTHESIA
N/A

WAKE UP AND EMERGENCE
N/A

ICU OR PACU
N/A

GI DISEASE

GEBHARD WAGENER, MD

SCREENING AND EVALUATION

Electrolytes
- Sodium: measure of volume status & dehydration
- Chloride: low w/ vomiting or diarrhea
- BUN, BUN/creatinine ratio: measure of dehydration
- Creatinine: impaired renal function? prerenal dehydration?
- Glucose extremely important: check bicarbonate to evaluate metabolic alkalosis, acidosis
- CBC: anemia? leukocytosis?

- Lactate: elevated: perforation, strangulation or sepsis?
- LFTs
- Coagulation profile
- Chest x-ray: position of diaphragm, basal atelectasis? air under diaphragm: perforation: left often gastric, right often duodenal or colonic?
- ECG
- Abdominal plain film: obstructive: air-fluid levels? free air? air/stool in rectum?
- Abdominal CT
- Echocardiogram: in intestinal ischemia: thrombus?

PREOPERATIVE PREPARATION
- Ensure adequate fluid resuscitation; pts are frequently severely dehydrated.
- Correct electrolyte abnormalities, esp. hypo- & hyperkalemia.

OPERATIVE PREPARATION
- Decompress stomach w/ orogastric or nasogastric tube.
- Abdominal CT
- Central venous catheter for evaluation of intravascular fluid status

ANESTHESIA
- Regional anesthesia almost always contraindicated
- Antibiotics prior to incision w/ anaerobic coverage
- Empty stomach & then remove gastric tube prior to induction of anesthesia.
- Generous fluid administration prior to induction to avoid postinduction hypotension; pts are frequently severely dehydrated (compensate for bowel prep) & do not tolerate vasodilation

Rapid sequence induction for:
- Obstructive intestinal diseases
- Gastroesophageal reflux disease
- Hiatal hernia

- Intestinal perforation
- Increased intra-abdominal pressure
- Motility disorders (eg, diabetic gastroparesis)

Prolonged pre-oxygenation required with increased intra-abdominal pressure: FRC low

In case of aspiration:

- Ventilate with $FiO_2 = 1.0$.
- Suction endotracheal tube.
- Consider fiberoptic bronchoscopy, especially w/ particulate aspiration.
- Prophylactic antibiotics or steroids not indicated

Avoid nitrous oxide:

- Intestinal gas volume is often increased in GI diseases (normal = 100 cc).
- Increase in intestinal gas volume can lead to bowel ischemia & perforation.
- Nitrous oxide accumulation already seen within 20 min after initiation

Adequate muscle relaxation allows best operating conditions for surgeon.

Abdominal surgery requires significantly more fluid administration to compensate for third-space loss (8–10 mL/kg/h).

WAKE UP AND EMERGENCE

- Empty stomach w/ nasogastric or orogastric tube prior to emergence.
- Ensure that pt is awake & has adequate airway reflexes: high risk for aspiration.

Neostigmine

- Increases intestinal motility (frequency & magnitude): parasympathomimetic: nausea, vomiting & rarely anastomosis breakdown
- Rule out pneumothorax prior to extubation if operation was near diaphragm: are breath sounds equal?

- Postop ventilation often required in pts receiving large amounts of IV fluids; increased intra-abdominal pressure decreases FRC.

ICU OR PACU
ICU admission for:
- Continued resuscitation
- Hemodynamic instability
- Sepsis, peritonitis
- Postop ventilation

Observe for increase in abdominal pressure (measure abdominal girth or bladder pressure).

Frequent hematocrit & hemoglobin measurements: rule out continued bleeding

For decreased urine output postop:
- Most frequently hypovolemia
- Rule out increased intra-abdominal pressure.
- Acute tubular necrosis possible: preoperative or intraoperative hypotension & renal hypoperfusion: check urine sodium
- Fluid resuscitation often required for at least 12–24 hrs postop: continued sequestration of fluid into bowel

---

HEMOGLOBINOPATHIES

DOUGLAS B. COURSIN, MD, AND KARL WILLMANN, MD

SCREENING AND EVALUATION
- CBC, Hgb not routinely acquired for most outpatients & many inpatients
- Identify high-risk pts (+ active or known history of anemia)
  - ➤ Obtain CBC
    - Determines WBC, Hct, Hgb, platelet count & indices
    - Reticulocyte count: bone marrow activity

PREOPERATIVE PREPARATION

- Identify anemia in high-risk pts or those undergoing high-risk surgery.
- Determine if anemia is of physiologic importance.
- Determine etiology:
  - ➤ Acute or chronic: Compensated or not?
  - ➤ If blood loss: Is it controlled? Does procedure need to be performed to control bleeding?
  - ➤ If secondary to nutrient deficiency: Does pt require supplementation (iron, vitamin B12, folate)? Is pt at risk for associated pathology? Neurologic disease w/ vitamin B12 deficiency? Abnormal homocysteine metabolism & folate?
  - ➤ Would the pt benefit from perioperative EPO?
    - Facilitate autologous predonation
    - Augment perioperative treatment of anemia
    - Available drugs: human recombinant EPO, darbopoietin
- Transfusion therapy
  - ➤ Based on acuity and severity of anemia, associated pathology, risk of surgery/procedure

OPERATIVE PREPARATION

- Address need for transfusion.
- Type & screen or cross-match if needed & not already performed.
- Determine availability of blood preop.

ANESTHESIA

- Maintain O_2 delivery.
  - ➤ Correct hypovolemia.
  - ➤ Avoid meds that depress cardiac function.
  - ➤ Avoid left shift in O_2 dissociation curve:
    - Avoid hypothermia (but may provide CNS protection).
    - Avoid acute alkalosis.
  - ➤ Avoid N_2O in pts w/ vitamin B12 or folate deficiencies.

➤ "Transfusion trigger" based on level of anemia, anticipated blood loss, individual reserve

WAKE UP AND EMERGENCE

■ Maintain O_2 delivery by maintaining good circulatory status
■ Treat shivering, excessive tachycardia or hypertension.

ICU OR PACU

■ > 50% of ICU pts are anemic within 72 hrs of ICU admission.
■ 1/7 ICU pts per day receive a transfusion in the ICU.
■ Over a third of all ICU pts receive transfusion during their ICU course.
■ Risk of transfusion increases with length of ICU stay.
■ Transfusions are independently associated w/ increased length of ICU stay, morbidity & mortality.
■ Increase transfusion trigger: CNS injury, myocardial ischemia or infarction

---

HEMOPHILIA A & HEMOPHILIA B

KARL WILLMANN, MD, & D. B. COURSIN, MD

SCREENING & EVALUATION

■ Schedule surgery early in the week so that special needs for laboratory & factor assays will be arranged for the preop, operative & postop time.
■ Hematologist consult prior to surgery

PREOPERATIVE PREPARATION

■ Factor levels drawn prior to surgery
■ IV access may difficult. Avoid IM injections.
■ Use invasive monitor only if necessary.

OPERATIVE PREPARATION

■ Hemophilia A: pts require a factor level 40–100%, depending on extent of surgery. These levels should be maintained 2–7 days postop, depending again on the extent of surgery. In large orthopedic surgeries, may need to maintain elevated factor VIII for several wks after surgery. Pts w/ mild to moderate disease may require only desmopressin (DDAVP); this drug can increase the level of activity of factor VIII 2–4x normal.

- Appropriate replacement of factors would be recombinant factor VIII.
- Elimination half-life of recombinant factor VIII is about 8 hrs.
- Dosing: 1 U/kg of recombinant factor VIII should increase plasma level of factor VIII by 0.02 U/mL, which is about a 2% increase in plasma activity.
- Pts who have had previous recombinant therapy may require recombinant factor VIIa if they have inhibitors to factor VIII (which occurs in 10–20%). This also is true for factor IX recombinant therapy.
- In emergencies, both cryoprecipitate & FFP could be used.
- Hemophilia B: pts should have levels of factor IX 30–75%, depending on extent of surgery. Replacement can be solvent/detergent-treated pooled factor IX & recombinant factor IX. Elimination half-life of recombinant therapy is about 24 hrs.
- Usual dose = body weight (kg) times desired factor IX increase (%) times 1.2 IU/kg. Maintain postop levels at 15–40%.
- Regional anesthesia: use w/ caution in light of pt's coagulopathy

ANESTHESIA
- Induction
  - ➤ Careful manipulation of airway to avoid bleeding
- Maintenance
  - ➤ No special concerns

WAKE UP & EMERGENCE
- Coughing & bucking on the endotracheal tube may lead to trauma of the airway & bleeding, causing airway compromise.

ICU OR PACU

- Avoid drugs that may impair clotting, such as NSAIDs, ASA & ketorolac.
- Monitor factor levels as necessary.

HERBAL THERAPY

JONATHAN T. KETZLER, MD

SCREENING & EVALUATION
N/A

PREOP PREPARATION
N/A

OPERATIVE PREPARATION
N/A

ANESTHESIA
N/A

WAKE UP & EMERGENCE
N/A

ICU OR PACU
N/A

HIV & AIDS

GEBHARD WAGENER, MD

SCREENING AND EVALUATION

History/exam

- Rx therapy: On HAART? How long?
- Pulmonary: Recent cough, fever
- Cardiac: Exercise tolerance?
- GI: Diarrhea, nausea, vomiting? Weight loss?

Investigations

■ Chest x-ray: Pneumonia? Pleural effusions?

■ ECG: Minimal voltage: Pleural effusion?

■ CD-4 count: CDC classification: grade 1, >499 normal, grade 2, 200–499; grade 3, <200/mcL (<50/mcL: high mortality)

■ WBC

■ Hct: anemia

■ Platelet count: HIV-induced thrombocytopenia

■ Echocardiogram: Pericardial effusion? LV function

■ PFT: restrictive disease secondary

■ Room air ABG

PREOPERATIVE PREPARATION

■ HIV does not increase perioperative mortality.

■ Treat pain adequately.

■ Do not avoid opioids w/ IV drug users.

OPERATIVE PREPARATION

■ Sterile technique for sterile procedures:
  ➤ Gown for central cannulations

■ Prophylactic antibiotics

■ Universal precautions!

■ In case of needlestick injury
  ➤ Wash out wound w/ iodine + alcohol-containing antiseptic.
  ➤ Report to employee health or emergency room immediately.
  ➤ Check HIV, hepatitis C, hepatitis B: health care worker, pt only with consent

■ Postexposure prophylaxis
  ➤ Zidovudine 250 mg BID
    • Lamivudine 150 mg BID
    • Indinavir 800 mg TID or nelfinavir 750 mg TID

■ Risk of infection: simple needlestick, 0.3–0.5%, w/ gloves 10–100x lower

ANESTHESIA

- Regional: preferable w/ pulmonary disease, but sterile technique!
- Epidural: probably higher incidence of catheter infections
- Document polyneuropathy (relative contraindication)
- Avoid succinylcholine w/ severe polyneuropathy.

WAKE UP AND EMERGENCE

- May be slowed w/ AIDS dementia
- Monitor neuromuscular blockade w/ polyneuropathy.

ICU OR PACU

- Depends on extent of surgery
- Mechanical ventilation for respiratory complications w/ PCP: high mortality

---

HYPERTENSION

MUHAMMED ITANI, MD, & JONATHAN T. KETZLER, MD

SCREENING AND EVALUATION

- History & physical exam: evaluate severity of symptoms, exercise tolerance
- EKG: acute ischemia, chronic LVH w/ strain, conduction disease
- CXR: cardiomegaly, pulmonary congestion/edema, pleural effusion
- TTE: LVH, dilated cardiomyopathy
- MRA: upper abdominal bruits (renovascular hypertension)
- Lab evaluation: end-organ damage, electrolyte disturbances
- Special studies
  - ➤ Pheochromocytoma: increased urinary vanillylmandelic & homovanillic acid
  - ➤ Conn's syndrome: high aldosterone, low renin

PREOPERATIVE PREPARATION

- Uncontrolled HTN
  - ➤ Delay elective surgery.
  - ➤ Admit for end-organ failure & treat.
- Continue antihypertensive meds until surgery.
  - ➤ Avoids rebound
  - ➤ Maintain intravascular volume.
- Normotension decreases the risk of the pt becoming hypotensive & developing ischemia intraoperatively.
- Hypertensive pts have a higher incidence of MI during surgery if they have a prior history of similar events & a higher incidence of stroke after carotid surgery.
- Do not stop clonidine & beta blockers; there is a high incidence of rebound hypertension; ACE inhibitors don't cause rebound hypertension if stopped preoperatively.
- ACE inhibitors can be kept the day before surgery if the surgery does not involve large fluid shifts & blood loss.
- Stop angiotensin II receptor blockers, as pts have a higher incidence of severe BP drops intraoperatively.

OPERATIVE PREPARATION

- Sedation may decrease anxiety in pts & thus control high BP preoperatively.
- Sedative requirements are reduced in pts on clonidine.
- Pts are hypovolemic, so adequate preop hydration can be important.
- Depending on the extent of cardiac disease, invasive monitors (CVP, arterial line) may be placed preoperatively.

ANESTHESIA

- Induction
  - ➤ Rapid-acting IV agents may be used for induction; dose & rapidity of introduction may be reduced due to the higher incidence of severe hypotension in these pts due to hypovolemia & peripheral vasodilation.

➤ Avoid ketamine because of potential to elevate BP markedly.

➤ Narcotics & inhalational anesthetics must be given to increase anesthetic depth before laryngoscopy is done to avoid sudden marked BP increase.

➤ Short-acting beta blockers (esmolol) may be used to acutely control increase in heart rate & BP w/ laryngoscopy.

➤ Fentanyl must be given in high doses (5–7 mcg/kg); inhalation agents should be given in 1.5 MAC doses to avoid cardiovascular response to intubation.

➤ Laryngoscopy should be done quickly (<15 sec).

➤ Lidocaine IV or intratracheal (1 mg/kg) may be used to attenuate the upper airway responses to intubation.

➤ If difficult or prolonged laryngoscopy is anticipated, IV nitroprusside or esmolol may be used for BP control.

➤ Take care to avoid hypotension because of all the above medication introduction.

■ Regional anesthesia is a safe option & helps avoid the BP swings seen w/ general anesthesia if limited sympathetic blockade is anticipated.

■ With central neuraxial blocks, severe drops in BP may be seen w/ chemical sympathectomies; aggressive fluid hydration may be done preop before the block is started to avoid this.

■ Maintenance

➤ Control the depth of anesthesia to avoid BP fluctuations.

➤ Adjust the depth so that surgical stimulation does not produce marked pressor response.

➤ Intraoperative hypotension is more common in pts whose BP was poorly controlled preoperatively.

➤ Response to surgical stimulation is exaggerated in pts w/ essential hypertension.

➤ Intraoperative hypotension can be controlled w/ fluid administration, sympathomimetics (phenylephrine, ephedrine) & decreasing the dose of inhalational agent.

➤ In surgeries involving sudden BP elevations (carotid surgery), vasodilator infusions (nitroprusside) may be prepared & used accordingly.

➤ In pts w/ regional anesthesia, use adequate sedation to avoid anxiety & subsequent hypotension.

➤ General anesthesia can be maintained using:
  • Volatile agents, low-solubility agents (sevoflurane, desflurane) may be preferred to highly soluble agents because of rapidity & ease of controlling depth of anesthesia.
  • N_2O/narcotic technique
  • No preference of one muscle relaxant over the other

■ Monitors
  ➤ Depends on extent of surgery & severity of disease
  ➤ 5-electrode EKG for myocardial ischemia detection
  ➤ Other standard ASA monitors
  ➤ Arterial line, PA catheter, CVP
  ➤ TEE w/ severe LV dysfunction

WAKE UP & EMERGENCE

■ Anxiety & pain control are very important to avoid hypertensive episodes.

■ Titrate narcotics to avoid oversedation.

■ May extubate at a deep level of anesthesia to avoid hypertensive response to upper airway instrumentation

■ Watch out for ischemic cardiac events (MI).

■ High risk of stroke w/ elevated BP

ICU OR PACU

■ Hypertension is common due to pain & relative hypovolemia.

■ Pain control is essential.

■ May continue monitors used intraoperatively in PACU

- If hypertension persists, can use hydralazine (2.5–10 mg q10–20min), nitroprusside (0.5–10 mcg/kg/min), labetalol (0.1–0.5 mg/kg q10min)
- Watch for hypertension-related complications:
  - Myocardial ischemia
  - Stroke
  - CHF
  - Dysrhythmias
  - Bleeding
- Pts w/ acute or ongoing target organ damage (subarachnoid hemorrhage postop, encephalopathy, CHF, renal insufficiency) may need immediate IV medication treatment in ICU setting; goal is gradual decrease in diastolic BP to avoid ischemia or infarction.
- Drop diastolic BP by 20% first hour; subsequent decrease should be achieved over 24–48 hrs.
- Nitroprusside IV: 0.5–10 mcg/kg/min; watch for cyanide poisoning.
- Hydralazine: watch for increase in ICP; may not be a choice in pts w/ neurologic disease
- Nitroglycerine: in hypertensive crisis secondary to myocardial ischemia or cocaine overdose
- Beta blockers: avoid w/ cocaine overdose

ICU PATIENT SCHEDULED FOR INTERCURRENT SURGERY

DOUGLAS B. COURSIN, MD

SCREENING AND EVALUATION
See "Overview" in the "Diseases" section.

PREOPERATIVE PREPARATION
- Full review of admission & ICU course
  - Attention to current meds, access, ventilatory needs
  - What is essential & what is not

➤ Continue or hold tube feedings.
➤ Continue or hold TPN.
  • If discontinued, follow glucose & evaluate for hypo-glycemia.
➤ Create ICU support & environment out of ICU in OR/cath lab, radiology suite.
■ Transport
■ Adequate equipment
  ➤ Adequate meds
  ➤ Adequate personnel
  ➤ Maintain normothermia.
  ➤ Maintain adequate ventilation.
    • Avoid under- or over-ventilation.
■ Consider starting anesthesia, at least analgesic & sedation (possibly neuromuscular paralysis), in ICU prior to transport, w/ careful observation of hemodynamic response.

OPERATIVE PREPARATION

■ Create ICU support & environment out of ICU in OR/cath lab, radiology suite.
■ Transport in & out of ICU location
  ➤ Adequate equipment
    • Adequate meds
    • Adequate personnel
    • Maintain normothermia.
    • Maintain adequate ventilation.
      • Avoid under- or over-ventilation.
■ Consider starting anesthesia, at least analgesic & sedation, in ICU prior to transport, w/ careful observation of hemody-namic response.
■ Maintain glucose control.
  ➤ Is pt on an insulin infusion? Is it w/ or w/out dextrose? Is it w/ or w/out potassium supplementation?
  ➤ If pt is not on an insulin infusion, is he or she likely to need one, depending on procedure & degree of stress hormone

response w/ insulin resistance & pro-inflammatory process, which may exacerbate hyperglycemia?
- Try to maintain glucose <150 mg/dL.
➤ Could the pt be relatively or absolutely adrenally insufficient?
- Does the pt need additional or stress dose of steroids?

ANESTHESIA
■ Titrate to effect.
■ Pt's hemodynamic reserve & response will dictate agents used & doses.
■ Requirements may be hard to predict, depending on pharmacodynamic & kinetic variables & presence of tolerance.
■ Aim for sedation, pain relief, amnesia & still pt.
■ Be prepared for hypotension secondary to induction, diminution of sympathetic nervous system, maintenance agents, patient positioning, ventilator requirements & operative technique.
■ Estimate & replace third-space losses.
■ Maintain normal temperature.
➤ Active/passive warming
➤ Blood warmers
➤ Low-flow or humidified gases
➤ Convection warmers
➤ If burn, warm room.
➤ If cold, actively warm.
➤ Fluid irrigation temperature

WAKE UP AND EMERGENCE
■ Do you want the pt to emerge? Transport while asleep?
■ Are you planning to extubate?
■ Is the pt going to PACU or ICU postop?
■ Can you adequately ventilate & support hemodynamically on transfer to PACU or ICU?
➤ What do you need to travel?

- Airway equipment, O_2, ventilatory, Ambu, resuscitation meds, current infusions

ICU OR PACU

- Most pts will return to ICU unless their primary process has been stabilized or reversed to a degree that would allow them to be transferred to an intermediate-care unit or floor bed.

- Key is to provide the same level of support as needed previously or escalated during the course of surgery or a procedure.

- Notify ICU of transfer so that ventilatory & hemodynamic support devices & meds are available on arrival.

- Consider transporting pt sedated & analgesed. If you plan extubation after the procedure, may be ideally suited to perform in ICU.

- Have adequate equipment, personnel, meds & O_2 to transfer back to ICU.

- On arrival, provide full report, particularly on intraoperative fluids, transfusions, antibiotics & any untoward events such as protracted hemodynamic changes or rhythm disturbances or exacerbations of gas exchange & surgical procedure.

- Outline postop plan:
  - Pain
  - Sedation
  - Ventilation
  - Hemodynamic control
  - Need for thermal regulation or support

IDIOPATHIC HYPERTROPHIC SUBAORTIC STENOSIS (IHSS)

ROBERT N. SLADEN, MD

SCREENING AND EVALUATION

- Note the following:
  - Symptoms (angina, syncope, congestive heart failure)

➤ Signs of progressive disease (ECG changes, valve gradient & area)
➤ Presence of associated CAD (increased risk)
■ Look for physical signs of:
  ➤ Left ventricular hypertrophy (apical heave)
  ➤ Congestive heart failure (elevated neck veins, edema, hepatomegaly)
■ Relevant lab studies
  ➤ Hct (anemia is poorly tolerated by low CO)
  ➤ PT, INR (if on coumadin for atrial fibrillation)
  ➤ BUN, creatinine (prerenal syndrome)
  ➤ ECG (LVH w/ or w/out strain)
  ➤ Chest x-ray (LVH)

PREOPERATIVE PREPARATION
■ Continue preop meds:
  ➤ Beta blockade or calcium blockade (negative inotropy, chronotropy)
  ➤ Digoxin (rate control for atrial fibrillation)
  ➤ Diuretics for pulmonary edema
■ Plan perioperative anticoagulation:
  ➤ Hold coumadin at least 3 days preop.
  ➤ Check INR prior to surgery.
■ Consider preop admission for control of:
  ➤ Rapid atrial fibrillation
  ➤ Symptomatic pulmonary edema or congestive heart failure
■ Plan perioperative antibiotics:
  ➤ Decrease risk of bacterial endocarditis

OPERATIVE PREPARATION
■ Review hemodynamic principles:
  ➤ Maintain sinus rhythm (atrial kick, to maximize ventricular filling).
  ➤ Maintain slow heart rate (increase diastolic fill time).
  ➤ Maintain adequate preload (maximize ventricular filling).

- ➤ Avoid inotropic, chronotropic agents.
- ➤ Avoid systemic vasodilators.
- ➤ Maintain SVR (& coronary diastolic perfusion pressure).
- ■ Acute (new-onset) atrial fibrillation
  - ➤ Poorly tolerated, can induce acute decompensation, low cardiac output syndrome
  - ➤ Treat aggressively whenever it occurs (esmolol, amiodarone, early cardioversion).
- ■ Ensure adequate sedative or opioid premedication
  - ➤ Suppress catecholamines, avoid tachyarrhythmias
  - ➤ BUT increased risk of respiratory depression (low cardiac output)
- ■ Use fluids & vasoconstrictor agents to treat hypotension
  - ➤ Maintain preload, diastolic perfusion pressure.
  - ➤ Avoid ephedrine, norepinephrine (mixed agonists, increase contractility, may induce tachycardia).
  - ➤ Use a pure vasoconstrictor (phenylephrine); reflex bradycardia is also helpful.
- ■ Invasive hemodynamic monitoring, TEE
  - ➤ Moderate to large fluid shifts anticipated
  - ➤ Presence of symptoms

ANESTHESIA
- ■ Regional anesthesia is relatively contraindicated
  - ➤ Sympathetic block may induce dangerous hypotension, worsen MVO_2
  - ➤ Avoid spinal anesthesia (abrupt onset of block).
  - ➤ Careful continuous spinal or epidural anesthesia may be tolerated.
  - ➤ Adequate fluid load prior to placement (maintain preload)
- ■ General anesthesia
  - ➤ Take measures to maintain slow heart rate & adequate perfusion pressure.
  - ➤ Preoxygenate

- ➤ Adequate fluid load prior to induction (maintain preload)
- ➤ Treat hypotension w/ phenylephrine.
- ➤ Treat tachycardia w/ esmolol.
- Avoid pancuronium (tachycardia), ketamine (sympathomimetic).
- Choose maintenance regimen that maintains slow heart rate, suppresses sympathetic response
  - ➤ Avoid isoflurane (increased heart rate), desflurane (increased sympathetic tone).
  - ➤ Consider sympatholytic opioid (fentanyl, sufentanil, remifentanil).

WAKE UP AND EMERGENCE
- Attempt to suppress catecholamines on emergence
  - ➤ Judicious use of sympatholytic opioid (fentanyl, sufentanil, remifentanil)
  - ➤ Avoid morphine (histamine, catecholamine release).
- Consider dexmedetomidine infusion
  - ➤ Sympatholytic, provides analgesia w/out respiratory depression
  - ➤ Can be continued through tracheal extubation & beyond
  - ➤ Dose carefully: can potentiate beta blockade, delay anesthetic emergence
- Potential complications on emergence
  - ➤ Delayed emergence (low cardiac output, increased pharmacodynamic effects)
  - ➤ Acute myocardial ischemia, pulmonary congestion, edema

ICU AND PACU
- Control pain & anxiety (avoid tachycardia); see above.
- Consider short period of postop mechanical ventilation if AS severe:
  - ➤ Allows controlled emergence

➤ Avoids reversal (ie, need for anticholinergic agents [tachycardia])

➤ Facilitates evaluation of cardiac, ventilatory function

➤ Careful sedation is essential: dexmedetomidine very useful

■ Restart preop meds (beta blockade, calcium blockade) as soon as possible.

ISCHEMIC HEART DISEASE

MUHAMMED ITANI, MD, AND JONATHAN T. KETZLER, MD

SCREENING & EVALUATION

■ History & physical exam

■ Risk factor assessment

■ Family history

■ 12-lead ECG

➤ May not show any abnormalities at rest or w/ no symptoms, or may show evidence of old MI (Q waves in 2 or more leads & >1/3 of the QRS complex length)

➤ May reveal ST segment depression >1 mm from baseline w/ angina pectoris or ST-segment elevation w/ AMI or variant angina

➤ Other changes w/ symptoms of angina pectoris: reversible T-wave inversion

➤ Other findings w/ AMI: increased T-wave amplitude, followed by ST elevation, followed by Q-wave development & resolution of ST elevation

■ Echocardiography can be used to assess global cardiac function. It can also be used to assess regional wall motion abnormalities & detect the presence of previous myocardial injury. LV function assessment is a major determinant of long-term prognosis. It is also used to diagnose LV thrombus in case of apical & anterior wall MI.

- Exercise electrocardiography is less accurate than imaging studies to establish diagnosis of IHD but can give an idea about LV function & prognosis. It may not be feasible in patients w/ severe PVD, limited exercise tolerance, paced rhythm, abnormal ST segment or aortic stenosis.
- Stress echocardiography is used w/ pharmacologic induction of cardiac stress (dobutamine) or exercise to look at LV segmental wall function at rest & w/ stress. This can be also used to differentiate between viable (hibernating, stunned) & nonviable (infarcted) myocardial segments. Echocardiography at rest can be used to assess LV function, which is an important prognostic variable.
- Nuclear stress imaging is used to assess coronary perfusion at rest & after stress. Nuclear tracers (technetium, thallium) are used to measure coronary blood flow.
- Positron emission tomography may be used to demonstrate regional myocardial blood flow & metabolism, & hence viability.
- Coronary angiography provides information about the coronary anatomy & the extent & location of the lesions. It is indicated in pts w/ unstable angina despite maximal therapy. It can provide a road map to coronary revascularization & the feasibility of percutaneous angioplasty or surgical treatment depending on the characteristics & location of the lesions.
- Cardiac enzyme elevation: CK, CK-MB & troponin (T & I). Troponin is more specific than CK-MB; increases within 4 hours after AMI & remains elevated up to 1 wk.

PREOPERATIVE PREPARATION
- ACC/AHA Guideline Update on Perioperative Cardiovascular Evaluation for Noncardiac Surgery can be used for risk stratification of patients w/ IHD. These guidelines can be found at the following link:
  http://www.americanheart.org/presenter.jhtml?identifier=3000370

- Risk stratification: assessment of the risk of development of cardiovascular complications perioperatively can be done based on:
  - ➤ Variables related to 4 major categories: nature of surgery (high, moderate or low risk), presence of IHD, presence of CHF & presence of cerebrovascular disease
  - ➤ Presence of comorbid conditions (diabetes mellitus, aortic stenosis, PVD)
  - ➤ Exercise tolerance
  - ➤ Studies may be ordered if disease severity has not been assessed previously.
- History & physical exam to assess extent of disease, exercise tolerance & symptom pattern, in addition to history of comorbid diseases
- Elective surgery in pts w/ a history of AMI should be delayed up to 6 months after the episode of AMI if possible. Intraoperative tachycardia can increase the risk of intraoperative ischemia & perioperative MI.
- Silent myocardial ischemia may be seen as only ECG changes w/ no history of symptoms. Almost 70–75% of ischemic episodes in IHD pts are silent, as well as 10–15% of AMIs.
- Continue beta blockers; they were found to increase long-term survival in patients w/ IHD.
- Calcium channel blockers do not increase the negative inotropic & vasodilatory effects of inhalational agents but may potentiate the effects of depolarizing & nondepolarizing muscle relaxants.
- Stop ACE inhibitors the night before surgery to avoid severe hypotension intraoperatively.
- Stop aspirin 1 wk before surgery if possible; anticoagulation must be held to decrease risk of bleeding.
- Patients w/ coronary stents should have their surgery delayed at least 4 wks after stenting when possible.
- Lifestyle modification may affect exercise tolerance (smoking cessation, diet).

- Cholesterol & triglyceride levels should be kept within acceptable range.
- Preop studies (ECG, chest x-ray, echocardiogram, etc.) may be indicated depending on risk stratification, IHD severity & disease progression.

OPERATIVE PREPARATION

- Minimizing the sympathetic system effects on the myocardium helps decrease the possibility of ischemic events perioperatively. This can be achieved by:
  - ➤ Anxiolysis w/ sedatives/narcotics (benzodiazepines, opioids, scopolamine 0.4–0.6 mg IM or 0.2–0.4 mg IV)
  - ➤ Continuation or administration of beta blockers
- Administration of nitroglycerine
- Maintain heart rate & blood pressure within 20% of normal values.

ANESTHESIA

- Induction
  - ➤ The main goal during induction is to avoid hypertension & tachycardia, thereby decreasing drastic cardiac events.
  - ➤ Minimize extreme variation in heart rate & blood pressure.
  - ➤ Avoid induction agents capable of stimulating sympathetic nervous system (ketamine, pancuronium).
  - ➤ Control cardiovascular response to tracheal intubation by keeping low duration of laryngoscopy (<15 sec) or by pharmacologic means. Pharmacologic interventions include lidocaine IV 1.5 to 2 min before intubation (1.5–2 mg/kg), intratracheal lidocaine (2 mg/kg) at the time of laryngoscopy, IV fentanyl 13 micrograms/kg, IV esmolol or IV nitroprusside.
  - ➤ Continuous nitroglycerine infusion was not found to decrease the incidence of intraoperative myocardial ischemia.

➤ Regional anesthesia may be preferred to general anesthesia if possible, as it tends to better block the stress response to surgery. Hypotension associated w/ some regional techniques should be corrected by fluids & sympathomimetic agents.

■ Maintenance

➤ Volatile anesthetics (isoflurane, desflurane & sevoflurane) are safe to use w/ IHD, provided severe CHF is not present.

➤ Alternative technique may be high-dose narcotic agent w/ oxygen & nitrous oxide.

➤ Avoid pancuronium to reduce sympathomimetic activity.

➤ Increased sensitivity to muscle relaxants may be seen in pts on calcium channel blockers.

➤ Keep BP & heart rate within 20% of awake values.

➤ Intraoperative ischemia may be treated with beta blockers (esmolol) in case of tachycardia, IV nitrates in the case of hypertension, or IV sympathomimetics & fluids w/ hypotension.

➤ Minimizing body heat loss is vital to avoid postop shivering & precipitation of ischemic myocardial events. This can be achieved w/ warm IV fluids, warm operating room atmosphere, forced warm air covers & irrigation of the surgical site w/ warm fluids.

➤ To maintain adequate myocardial oxygen delivery, do not allow hemoglobin to drop below 10 g/dL.

■ Monitors used depend on disease severity & operative procedure complexity.

➤ ECG: simplest & most commonly used. ST-segment changes are principally used to diagnose myocardial ischemia. ST-segment analysis should be used for accurate determination of ST-segment changes. Most commonly used leads are II & V5, since these reflect ischemic changes in RCA & LAD distributions, respectively.

➤ Pulmonary artery catheter: ischemia manifests as a sudden increase in PCWP, in addition to new V waves in case of new onset of ischemic mitral valve regurgitation. This may not be seen w/ small areas of ischemia. PA diastolic pressure is less sensitive to ischemic changes. Since PCWP is measured intermittently, it may be more valuable in guiding treatment than detection of ischemia (fluids & medication administration, & measuring changes in myocardial function & systemic vascular resistance).

➤ Central venous pressure may correlate w/ PCWP if EF = 0.5 & there is no evidence of LV dysfunction.

➤ Transesophageal echocardiography: most sensitive to detect intraoperative myocardial ischemia by detecting new onset of regional wall motion abnormality

WAKE UP AND EMERGENCE

■ Proper pain control is key to avoid myocardial ischemic events.

■ Muscle relaxants can be reversed w/ neostigmine in combination w/ glycopyrrolate, as the latter produces less tachycardia. Nevertheless, atropine can be used w/ no adverse effects as long as the pt is adequately beta blocked.

■ Continuous ECG monitoring w/ ST-segment analysis is important to detect any myocardial ischemic events.

■ Supplemental oxygen to maintain adequate oxygen saturation is important.

■ Adequate heart rate & BP control as intraoperatively

■ Treat tachycardia or hemodynamic instability.

■ Avoid & treat shivering.

ICU OR PACU

■ Supplemental oxygen is crucial.

■ Pain control to avoid excessive sympathetic nervous system stimulation

- Maintain adequate beta blockade.
- 12-lead ECG as a baseline
- Prevention of shivering & maintenance of normothermia is crucial to avoid oxygen desaturation & sympathetic nervous system activation.
- Troponin levels q8h 3x postop, specifically after major vascular surgery. In pts w/ values 1.5 or above, mortality 6 months postop may be higher than those w/ lower values.
- Maintaining adequate oxygenation & tight pain control for 48 to 72 hr postop is very important, since this is the period when the likelihood of developing AMI is highest.
- Reasonable control of blood glucose: keep blood glucose levels 100–180 mg/dL.

LATEX ALLERGY

ARTHUR ATCHABAHIAN, MD

SCREENING AND EVALUATION

- Biological testing includes RAST (radioallergosorbent testing), but specificity & sensitivity are questionable.
- Use tests (wearing a latex glove) or skin prick more reliable, but risk of serious reaction including anaphylaxis
- It is preferable to treat any at-risk pt as having demonstrated latex allergy.

PREOPERATIVE PREPARATION

- First patient in operating room
- Surgical, operating room & PACU/ICU staff alerted
- A latex-free kit containing safe supplies should be available.
- Question any equipment to be used around the pt.
- Steroids/antihistamine pretreatment has not been shown to be helpful.

OPERATIVE PREPARATION

■ Remove any latex-containing equipment while wearing vinyl gloves, then discard gloves.

■ Place signs on door to prevent entrance of outside personnel potentially carrying latex particles.

■ Remove rubber stopper on vials with a clamp prior to drawing meds (although most do not contain latex).

■ Use green latex-free bag on anesthesia machine (in latex-free kit).

■ Use vinyl gloves & non-latex tourniquet (in latex-free kit).

■ Surgical team should use latex-free sterile gloves (neoprene, PVC or other).

■ Use PVC NIBP cuff or protect skin with Soffban (in latex-free kit).

■ Do not use Elastoplast or fabric tape.

■ Do not use injection ports on IV tubing, IV bags & burettes; place tape over them; inject meds or draw fluid through 3-way stopcock.

■ Ensure that kits (spinal, epidural, etc.) are latex-free; specifically, some syringes contain latex.

■ Be fully prepared to treat bronchospasm and/or anaphylaxis.

ANESTHESIA

■ Use clear face masks, not black rubber masks.

■ Do not use red rubber ETTs.

■ All LMAs are safe.

■ Inject meds or draw fluid through 3-way stopcock; do not use injection ports.

■ Use silicone Foley catheter.

■ Do not use Swan-Ganz catheter (balloon contains latex).

WAKE UP AND EMERGENCE

■ Unremarkable

ICU OR PACU

- Single (isolation) room to prevent exposure to latex particles
- If possible, one nurse for pt
- Similar precautions for monitoring equipment & medication/fluid administration
- If not previously done, counsel pt & family.
- Bracelet indicating latex allergy
- Allergist consultation
- Pt should carry self-injecting epinephrine syringe.

LIVER DISEASE

ROBERT N. SLADEN, MD

SCREENING & EVALUATION

- Signs of hepatocellular failure
  - Spider nevi, palmar erythema, Dupuytren's contracture
  - Gynecomastia, testicular atrophy, loss of body hair
  - Anasarca, ecchymoses, anemia, malnutrition
- Signs of portal hypertension
  - Ascites, splenomegaly
  - Caput medusae (engorged veins around umbilicus)
- Relevant lab studies
  - Hct, CBC, prothrombin time
  - Electrolytes (total CO_2 if ABG impracticable)
  - BUN, creatinine
  - LFTs, arterial ammonia
  - ECG & chest x-ray
- Child-Pugh classification of preoperative risk in cirrhosis
  - A: low risk (<10% mortality)
  - B: moderate risk (5–20% mortality)
  - C: high risk (up to 75% mortality)
- Components of score

- ➤ Jaundice (serum bilirubin)
- ➤ Hypoalbuminemia (serum albumin)
- ➤ PT, seconds > control
- ➤ Encephalopathy
- ➤ Ascites
- ➤ Nutrition
- ■ Child's A
  - ➤ Serum bilirubin < 2 mg/dL
  - ➤ Serum albumin > 3.5 mg/dL
  - ➤ PT 1–4 seconds > control
  - ➤ Encephalopathy grade 0
  - ➤ Ascites absent
  - ➤ Nutrition excellent
- ■ Child's B
  - ➤ Serum bilirubin 2–3 mg/dL
  - ➤ Serum albumin 3–3.5 mg/dL
  - ➤ PT 4–6 seconds > control
  - ➤ Encephalopathy grade 1–2
  - ➤ Ascites, easily controlled
  - ➤ Nutrition good
- ■ Child's C
  - ➤ Serum bilirubin > 3 mg/dL
  - ➤ Serum albumin < 3 mg/dL
  - ➤ PT >6 seconds > control
  - ➤ Encephalopathy grade 3–4
  - ➤ Ascites, difficult to control
  - ➤ Nutrition poor

PREOPERATIVE PREPARATION
- ■ Postpone elective surgery (high morbidity & mortality):
  - ➤ Acute viral hepatitis, Child's C
  - ➤ PT remains >3 sec > control despite parenteral vitamin K and/or FFP
- ■ Hepatorenal syndrome

- ➤ Discontinue spironolactone 3–4 days preop (promotes K retention).
- ➤ Cautiously drain tense ascites.
- ➤ Consider TIPS (see below).
- ■ Treat & remove precipitating factors of encephalopathy:
  - ➤ Protein restriction, lactulose, neomycin
- ■ Acute GI bleeding
  - ➤ Fluid resuscitation, transfusion, correction of coagulopathy
  - ➤ Establish diagnosis (varices vs. peptic ulcer)
  - ➤ Refractory bleeding options: transjugular intrahepatic portasystemic shunt (TIPS), endoscopic sclerotherapy, Sengstaken-Blakemore tube (w/ or w/out tracheal intubation), vasopressin infusion, emergency decompression
- ■ TIPS
  - ➤ Decompresses portal hypertension, relieves ascites, improves renal function, decreases risk of endotoxemia, pulmonary edema, encephalopathy

OPERATIVE PREPARATION
- ■ Minimize sedative or opioid premed.
  - ➤ If necessary, give small doses of IV sedation in induction room or OR under direct observation.
- ■ Aspiration prophylaxis
  - ➤ Anticholinergic agent (glycopyrrolate preferred)
  - ➤ H2 blocker (famotidine preferred)
  - ➤ Metoclopramide
  - ➤ Sodium bicitrate
- ■ Use universal & aseptic precautions throughout.
  - ➤ All staff should have hepatitis B vaccine.
- ■ Invasive hemodynamic monitoring
  - ➤ If large fluid shifts anticipated
  - ➤ High risk of perioperative acute renal failure (hepatorenal syndrome)

➤ Intravascular volume status difficult to assess (ascites & anasarca)
■ Careful positioning
  ➤ Fragile skin, easy bruising
  ➤ Tense ascites (discomfort, respiratory compromise)
■ Use active warming devices to prevent hypothermia:
  ➤ Forced-air convection blanket

ANESTHESIA
■ Regional anesthesia
  ➤ Preserves hepatic blood flow (HBF) if BP, cardiac output maintained
  ➤ Usually not practicable (coagulopathy, ascites)
■ General anesthesia
  ➤ Drug handling is extremely variable.
  ➤ Alcoholics require large loading doses; elimination & emergence delayed
  ➤ Decrease doses of all sedative/anesthetic agents in severe liver disease.
■ Anesthetic induction
  ➤ Aspiration precautions (head up, rapid sequence, cricoid pressure)
  ➤ Preoxygenate
  ➤ Adequate fluid load (250–1,000 mL) prior to induction
■ Neuromuscular blockade
  ➤ Succinylcholine duration can be prolonged (low pseudo-cholinesterase).
  ➤ Atracurium, cisatracurium preferred (elimination independent of liver function)
■ Choice of anesthetic agents
  ➤ All volatile anesthetic agents decrease HBF.
  ➤ All opioids may accumulate.
  ➤ Propofol remains relatively short-acting in cirrhosis.

- Avoid hypercarbia, hypocarbia (cause portal constriction, decrease HBF).
  - ➤ Anticipate intraoperative complications:
    - Hypoxemia (ascites, shunting)
    - Bleeding (coagulopathy)
    - Oliguria (vasomotor nephropathy)
  - ➤ Renal protection used in hepatorenal syndrome (prophylaxis not evidence-based):
    - Dopamine (use as diuretic and/or inotropic agent)
    - Furosemide infusion
    - Fenoldopam (selective DA-1 dopaminergic agonist)
- Excessive volume loading can induce acute hepatic congestion:
  - ➤ Fluid restriction decreases venous oozing, bleeding.
  - ➤ Keep CVP <10 mm Hg if possible.
  - ➤ Defer fluid resuscitation until after hepatic resection.

WAKE UP & EMERGENCE

- Anesthetic emergence may be delayed.
- Potential complications on emergence
  - ➤ Vomiting, aspiration
  - ➤ Hypotension
  - ➤ Persistent neuromuscular blockade
  - ➤ Respiratory depression
  - ➤ Acute respiratory failure
- Extubate trachea when pt fully awake.

ICU & PACU

- Consider short period of postop mechanical ventilation:
  - ➤ Allows controlled emergence
  - ➤ Facilitates evaluation of neurologic, ventilatory function
- Anticipate postop complications:
  - ➤ Bleeding & refractory coagulopathy
  - ➤ Oliguria & acute renal failure
  - ➤ Encephalopathy

- Acute respiratory failure
- Sepsis & wound dehiscence
- Acute hepatic failure
- Chronic hepatic insufficiency (ascites, jaundice, malnutrition, "failure to thrive")

MALIGNANT HYPERTHERMIA

HUGH R. PLAYFORD, MD

SCREENING AND EVALUATION

History
- Previous anesthetics & specific agents
- Family history (inheritance may be autosomal dominant, autosomal recessive or multifactorial, or unclassified). Penetrance may be incomplete.
- Associated conditions (see "Malignant Hyperthermia" in the "Diseases" section)

Exam
- Usually normal
- May have evidence of associated conditions

Investigations
- Open muscle biopsy & contractile testing
  - Susceptible (abnormal response to both halothane & caffeine)
  - Equivocal (abnormal response to either halothane or caffeine)
  - Normal (no response)
- Chromosomal testing: 19q (limited sensitivity & specificity)
- Other (lymphocyte & platelet tests): less useful

PREOPERATIVE PREPARATION
- Goal is to reduce triggering episode.

- Plan to be in an environment able to treat MH crisis (if needed).

OPERATIVE PREPARATION
- Remove or bypass vaporizers.
- Replace fresh gas outlet hose, breathing system tubing, carbon dioxide absorbent.
- Flush machine (>10 min at 10 L/min, if unable to remove fresh gas outlet hose >20 min at 10 L/min).
- Bain circuit acceptable for non-crisis anesthesia (circle for crisis)
- Dantrolene availability for all
- Dantrolene prophylaxis is controversial. Consider for pts:
  - ➤ W/ limited cardiac & cerebrovascular reserve
  - ➤ Unable to tolerate hypermetabolism
  - ➤ W/ history of awake stress-induced MH
  - ➤ Dose 2.5 mg/kg IV at induction, 1.25 mg/kg IV/PO q6h for 2–3 days

ANESTHESIA
Avoid triggering agents:
- Succinylcholine, volatile anesthetics (halothane, enflurane, isoflurane, sevoflurane, desflurane)

Use non-triggering agents:
- IV induction agents (barbiturates, propofol, benzodiazepines, ketamine, droperidol)
- Narcotics & nitrous oxide
- Nondepolarizing neuromuscular blockers
- Local anesthetics (amides now seen as safe)
- Anticholinesterases & anticholinergics
- Catecholamines, digoxin, calcium

Monitoring (dictated by comorbidity)
- NIBP, ECG, pulse oximetry, capnometry, temperature

WAKE UP AND EMERGENCE

Anticholinesterases & anticholinergics regarded as safe

ICU OR PACU

PACU

■ Monitor temperature for 4 hrs (if normal, discharge to floor or home).

ICU if:

■ MH crisis

■ Surgical or comorbidity require

MITRAL REGURGITATION

ROBERT N. SLADEN, MD

SCREENING AND EVALUATION

■ Note the following:
  ➤ History of atrial fibrillation
  ➤ Symptoms of pulmonary edema (ie, dyspnea, hemoptysis, orthopnea)
  ➤ Symptoms of congestive heart failure (ie, weight gain, edema, anasarca)

■ Look for physical signs of:
  ➤ Atrial fibrillation
  ➤ Pulmonary edema (orthopnea, crackles)
  ➤ Congestive heart failure (elevated neck veins, edema, hepatomegaly)
  ➤ Cardiac cachexia, "malar flush"

■ Relevant lab studies
  ➤ Hct (anemia of chronic disease)
  ➤ PT, INR (reversal of coumadin effect)
  ➤ BUN, creatinine (prerenal syndrome)
  ➤ ECG (atrial fibrillation)

➤ Chest x-ray (left atrial & ventricular enlargement, pulmonary edema)

PREOPERATIVE PREPARATION
- Continue preop meds:
  - ➤ Digoxin (rate control for atrial fibrillation)
  - ➤ Diuretics for pulmonary edema
- Plan perioperative anticoagulation:
  - ➤ Hold coumadin at least 3 days preoperatively.
  - ➤ Check INR before surgery.
- Consider preop admission for control of:
  - ➤ Rapid atrial fibrillation
  - ➤ Symptomatic pulmonary edema or congestive heart failure
- Plan perioperative antibiotics:
  - ➤ Decrease risk of bacterial endocarditis

OPERATIVE PREPARATION
- Review hemodynamic principles:
  - ➤ Maintain sinus rhythm (atrial kick, to maximize ventricular filling)
  - ➤ Maintain faster heart rate (increase forward cardiac output)
  - ➤ Maintain adequate preload (maximize ventricular filling)
  - ➤ Use inotropic, chronotropic agents (maintain forward ejection, faster heart rate)
  - ➤ Provide afterload reduction w/ systemic vasodilators (increase forward fraction of ejection)
- Control pulmonary hypertension:
  - ➤ Avoid hypoxemia, hypercarbia, acidosis (induce pulmonary vasoconstriction)
  - ➤ Use balanced vasodilators (nitroprusside)
  - ➤ Severe: consider inhaled prostacyclin, inhaled nitric oxide
- Acute (new-onset) atrial fibrillation

- ➤ Poorly tolerated, can induce acute decompensation, pulmonary edema
- ➤ Treat aggressively whenever it occurs (esmolol, amiodarone, early cardioversion)
- Ensure adequate sedative or opioid premedication:
  - ➤ Suppress catecholamines, avoid tachyarrhythmias
  - ➤ But increased risk of respiratory depression (low cardiac output)
- Consider perioperative vasodilation w/ nitroprusside (balanced vasodilator)
  - ➤ Provides preload & afterload reduction
- Use fluids & inotropic agents to treat hypotension
  - ➤ Maintain preload, contractility
  - ➤ Ephedrine may be useful (mixed agonist, increases contractility, induces tachycardia)
  - ➤ Excessive vasoconstriction (phenylephrine, norepinephrine) may increase regurgitation.
- Invasive hemodynamic monitoring
  - ➤ Large fluid shifts anticipated
  - ➤ Rapid changes in afterload anticipated (may lead to rapid changes in regurgitant fraction)
  - ➤ Presence of pulmonary congestion/edema or congestive heart failure

ANESTHESIA
- Regional anesthesia
  - ➤ Precautions w/ prior coumadin therapy (avoid if INR still >1.4)
  - ➤ Sympathetic blockade (vasodilation, afterload reduction) can markedly improve regurgitation.
  - ➤ Adequate fluid load before placement (maintain preload)
  - ➤ Systemic hypotension may induce low cardiac output.
  - ➤ Beware of postop pulmonary edema (sympathetic block wears off, increase in SVR).

- General anesthesia
  - ➤ Pt may not tolerate lying flat (orthopnea).
  - ➤ Take measures to maintain heart rate, contractility (eg, dopamine, dobutamine).
  - ➤ Preoxygenate
  - ➤ Adequate fluid load before induction (maintain preload)
- Avoid nitrous oxide
  - ➤ Exacerbates underlying pulmonary hypertension
- Choose maintenance regimen that does not depress myocardium, induce bradycardia
  - ➤ Avoid halothane, enflurane.
  - ➤ Consider total IV anesthesia w/ opioid (fentanyl, sufentanil, remifentanil).

WAKE UP AND EMERGENCE

- Attempt to suppress catecholamines on emergence (tachyarrhythmias)
  - ➤ Judicious use of sympatholytic opioid (fentanyl, sufentanil, remifentanil)
  - ➤ Avoid morphine (histamine, catecholamine release).
- Potential complications on emergence
  - ➤ Delayed emergence (low cardiac output, increased pharmacodynamic effects)
  - ➤ Acute pulmonary hypertension
  - ➤ Acute pulmonary congestion, edema
  - ➤ Hypoxemia, acute respiratory failure

ICU AND PACU

- Maintain cardiac output
  - ➤ Maintain preload (fluids).
  - ➤ Aggressive treatment of atrial arrhythmias (esmolol, amiodarone, cardioversion)
  - ➤ Maintain or increase contractility (dopamine).
  - ➤ Decrease afterload w/ vasodilators (nitroprusside, nicardipine).

➤ Increase contractility, decrease afterload with inodilators (dobutamine, milrinone).
■ Consider short period of postop mechanical ventilation if MR severe
  ➤ Allows controlled emergence
  ➤ Avoids reversal (ie, need for muscarinic agents [bradycardia])
  ➤ Facilitates evaluation of cardiac, ventilatory function
  ➤ Allows control of pulmonary hypertension, appropriate diuresis before extubation
■ Restart preop meds (digoxin, diuretics) as soon as possible.
■ For chronic atrial fibrillation
  ➤ Anticoagulation required >24 hr to prevent intracardiac thrombus formation
  ➤ Restart oral coumadin when able to take orally.
  ➤ If not, start IV heparin & continue until able to take oral meds.

MITRAL STENOSIS

ROBERT N. SLADEN, MD

SCREENING AND EVALUATION
■ Note the following:
  ➤ History of atrial fibrillation
  ➤ Symptoms of pulmonary edema (ie, dyspnea, hemoptysis, orthopnea)
■ Look for physical signs of:
  ➤ Atrial fibrillation
  ➤ Pulmonary edema (orthopnea, crackles)
  ➤ Cardiac cachexia, "malar flush"
■ Relevant lab studies
  ➤ Hct (anemia of chronic disease)

➤ PT, INR (reversal of coumadin effect)

➤ BUN, creatinine (prerenal syndrome)

➤ ECG (atrial fibrillation)

➤ Chest x-ray (left atrial enlargement, pulmonary edema)

PREOPERATIVE PREPARATION

■ Continue preop meds:

➤ Digoxin (rate control for atrial fibrillation)

➤ Diuretics for pulmonary edema

■ Plan perioperative anticoagulation:

➤ Hold coumadin at least 3 days preop.

➤ Check INR before surgery.

■ Consider preop admission for control of:

➤ Rapid atrial fibrillation

➤ Symptomatic pulmonary edema

■ Plan perioperative antibiotics:

➤ Decrease risk of bacterial endocarditis

OPERATIVE PREPARATION

■ Review hemodynamic principles:

➤ Maintain sinus rhythm (atrial kick, to overcome mitral gradient).

➤ Maintain slow heart rate (increases diastolic fill time for ventricle).

➤ Avoid tachycardia (promotes pulmonary hypertension, edema).

➤ Maintain adequate preload (overcome mitral gradient).

➤ Avoid inotropic, chronotropic agents (no benefit to left ventricle).

➤ Avoid systemic vasodilators (afterload reduction is of no benefit).

■ Control pulmonary hypertension:

➤ Avoid hypoxemia, hypercarbia, acidosis (induce pulmonary vasoconstriction)

➤ Use venodilators (nitroglycerin)

- ➤ Severe: consider inhaled prostacyclin, inhaled nitric oxide
- ▪ Acute (new-onset) atrial fibrillation
  - ➤ Poorly tolerated; can induce acute decompensation, pulmonary edema
  - ➤ Treat aggressively whenever it occurs (esmolol, early cardioversion).
- ▪ Ensure adequate sedative or opioid premedication:
  - ➤ Suppress catecholamines, avoid tachycardia
  - ➤ But increased risk of respiratory depression (low cardiac output)
- ▪ Consider titratable beta blockade (esmolol) for rate control.
- ▪ Consider perioperative venodilation w/ nitroglycerin (selective venodilator):
  - ➤ Avoid sodium nitroprusside (arterial hypotension).
- ▪ Choose an appropriate vasoconstrictor to treat hypotension:
  - ➤ Use phenylephrine (pure alpha agonist, induces reflex bradycardia).
  - ➤ Avoid ephedrine (mixed agonist, induces tachycardia).
- ▪ Invasive hemodynamic monitoring
  - ➤ Large fluid shifts anticipated
  - ➤ Presence of pulmonary congestion or edema

ANESTHESIA
- ▪ Regional anesthesia
  - ➤ Precautions w/ prior coumadin therapy (avoid if INR still >1.4)
  - ➤ Sympathetic blockade is helpful in controlling pulmonary congestion, edema
  - ➤ Adequate fluid load before placement (maintain preload)
  - ➤ Systemic hypotension, reflex tachycardia may induce low cardiac output, pulmonary hypertension.
  - ➤ Beware of postop pulmonary edema (sympathetic block wears off, increase in SVR).

- General anesthesia
  - Pt may not tolerate lying flat (orthopnea).
  - Take measures to control tachycardia (eg, esmolol, remifentanil).
  - Preoxygenate.
- Adequate fluid load before induction (maintain preload)
- Avoid pancuronium (tachycardia), ketamine (sympathomimetic).
- Avoid nitrous oxide:
  - Exacerbates underlying pulmonary hypertension
- Choose maintenance regimen that maintains slow heart rate, suppresses sympathetic response:
  - Avoid isoflurane (increased heart rate), desflurane (increased sympathetic tone).
  - Consider sympatholytic opioid (fentanyl, sufentanil, remifentanil).

WAKE UP AND EMERGENCE
- Attempt to suppress catecholamines on emergence:
  - Judicious use of sympatholytic opioid (fentanyl, sufentanil, remifentanil)
  - Avoid morphine (histamine, catecholamine release).
- Consider dexmedetomidine infusion:
  - Sympatholytic, provides analgesia w/out respiratory depression
  - Can be continued through tracheal extubation & beyond
  - Dose carefully: can potentiate beta blockade, delay anesthetic emergence
- Potential complications on emergence
  - Delayed emergence (low cardiac output, increased pharmacodynamic effects)
  - Acute pulmonary hypertension
  - Acute pulmonary congestion, edema

➤ Hypoxemia, acute respiratory failure

ICU AND PACU
- Control pain & anxiety (avoid tachycardia); see above.
- Consider short period of postop mechanical ventilation if severe disease:
  ➤ Allows controlled emergence
  ➤ Avoids reversal (ie, need for anticholinergic agents [tachycardia])
  ➤ Facilitates evaluation of cardiac, ventilatory function
  ➤ Allows control of pulmonary hypertension, appropriate diuresis before extubation
- Restart preop meds (digoxin, diuretics) as soon as possible.
- For chronic atrial fibrillation
  ➤ Anticoagulation required >24 hr to prevent intracardiac thrombus formation
  ➤ Restart oral coumadin when pt is able to take orally.
  ➤ If not, start IV heparin & continue until pt is able to take oral meds.

MORBID OBESITY

HUGH R. PLAYFORD, MD

SCREENING AND EVALUATION
- Note the following:
  ➤ Previous anesthesia (difficulty w/ intubation or airway maintenance, nerve blocks, positioning)
  ➤ Obesity hypoventilation syndrome, Pickwickian syndrome
  ➤ Esophageal reflux
  ➤ Obesity meds
    • Sibutramide (hypertension, serotonin syndrome)
    • Fenfluramine-phenteramine (withdrawn from market, cardiac valve defects)

- Look for physical signs of:
  - ➤ Hypertension, L or R ventricular failure, pulmonary hypertension
  - ➤ Limited mouth opening, limited neck movement, intra-oral soft tissues
- Relevant lab studies
  - ➤ Hct, CBC
  - ➤ Serum biochemistry (incl. glucose, LFTs)
  - ➤ ABGs on room air (hypoxemia [increased metabolic rate, V/Q mismatch], normocarbia)
  - ➤ ECG, chest x-ray
  - ➤ W/ or w/out echo
  - ➤ Pulmonary function tests (usually restrictive pattern w/ decreased ERV, VC, FRC & tidal volume, increased RR)

PREOPERATIVE PREPARATION

- CPAP/BiPAP
  - ➤ Continue to time of surgery.
  - ➤ Ensure available immediately postop for wake up/emergence/PACU/postop course.
- Reflux meds
  - ➤ Continue to time of surgery.
- Glucose intolerance
  - ➤ Manage as per diabetic routine (fasting, hypoglycemics, Dextrostix, timing of surgery).

OPERATIVE PREPARATION

- Avoid respiratory depressants until in OR.
- Avoid subcutaneous or intramuscular routes (unpredictable absorption).
- Anti-sialogogue if awake intubation considered
- Gastric regurgitation precautions (decreased volume, increased pH)

➤ H2 receptor antagonist, gastric prokinetic, gastric tube
- Appropriate equipment for obese pts
  ➤ Operating tables, gurneys
  ➤ Padding of pressure points

ANESTHESIA
- Monitoring & equipment
  ➤ Blood pressure
    • NIBP (w/ appropriate cuff size)
    • Invasive arterial monitoring
  ➤ ECG (II, aVF, V5 for cardiac ischemia)
  ➤ Other invasive monitoring as indicated (pulmonary artery catheters, echo)
  ➤ Respiratory parameters
    • SaO_2, w/ or w/out ABGs
    • $EtCO_2$
  ➤ Peripheral nerve stimulator (w/ or w/out needle electrodes)
  ➤ Temperature (prevent hypothermia, shivering, subsequent hypoxia)
    • Monitoring
    • Forced-air warmers
- Airway mgt
  ➤ For general anesthesia, consider endotracheal tube
    • Difficult mask ventilation
    • High risk of gastric aspiration
    • Obese pts tend to spontaneously hypoventilate (hypoxia, hypercarbia, acidosis).

WAKE UP AND EMERGENCE
N/A

ICU OR PACU
N/A

MULTIPLE SCLEROSIS

KARL WILLMANN, MD

SCREENING AND EVALUATION

- Neurologic evaluation
  - Duration of MS signs & symptoms
  - Bulbar dysfunction
  - Respiratory dysfunction (CXR ± PFTs, ABGs)
  - Peripheral signs (particularly if considering regional anesthesia)
- Toxicity of pharmacotherapy
  - Preop EKG, CBC & renal function tests
  - IVIG, interferon beta 1-a (Avonex), interferon beta 1-b (Betaseron), glatiramer acetate (Copaxone) & mitoxantrone (Novantrone) may cause marrow suppression, renal failure, arrhythmias, seizures & cardiac arrest.
- Anesthetic considerations
  - Paraplegia/quadriplegia: risk of autonomic hyperreflexia
  - Pharyngeal & laryngeal muscular impairment: risk of aspiration

PREOPERATIVE PREPARATION

- Aspiration precautions (esp. w/ pharyngeal/laryngeal dysfunction)
  - Metoclopramide (Reglan), H_2 blocker, or
  - Proton pump inhibitor, or
  - Non-particulate antacids
- Continue MS meds until time of surgery.

OPERATIVE PREPARATION

- Arterial line
  - Pulmonary dysfunction
  - Paraplegia, quadriplegia
  - History or risk of autonomic hyperreflexia
- Urinary catheter

➤ Minimize autonomic responses to bladder distention
■ Temperature monitoring
  ➤ Exacerbation of MS weakness is associated w/ hyperthermia.
  ➤ Avoid hyperthermia & treat aggressively if it develops.
■ Positioning
  ➤ Care w/ sensory deficits, spasticity, paraplegia, quadriplegia
  ➤ IV & line placement may be difficult.

ANESTHESIA
■ Induction w/ aspiration precautions (pharyngeal, laryngeal dysfunction)
  ➤ Rapid sequence induction
  ➤ Preoxygenation + cricothyroid pressure + head up
  ➤ Avoid succinylcholine (potential for exaggerated K release).
■ Maintenance
  ➤ Regional/neuraxial anesthesia
    • May cause exacerbation of MS (but no prospective evidence)
    • No reported exacerbation of MS w/ epidural for labor pain
    • Not contraindicated if GA poses a greater risk than regional

WAKE UP AND EMERGENCE
■ Anticipate delayed emergence:
  ➤ Anesthetics (benzodiazepines potentiate)
  ➤ Non-depolarizing neuromuscular blockers
    • Baclofen (Lioresal)
    • Dantrolene (Dantrium)
    • Propantheline (Pro-Banthine)
■ Anticipate pulmonary compromise:
  ➤ Ensure pts are awake, fully reversed from neuromuscular blockade

➤ Able to maintain good oxygenation & ventilation
➤ Do not extubate if above criteria not met.
■ Anticipate potential for pulmonary aspiration.

ICU OR PACU
■ Consider a period of postop ventilation & ICU care:
➤ Severe pulmonary compromise
■ Thoracic/abdominal procedures

MUSCULAR DYSTROPHY

JONATHAN T. KETZLER, MD

SCREENING AND EVALUATION
■ Necrotic & phagocytized muscle fibers are seen on biopsy.
■ Levels of serum enzymes derived from muscle tissue (creatinine kinase, lactate dehydrogenase, aspartate aminotransferase, alanine aminotransferase) & myoglobin usually correlate with severity of disease.
■ Do a pulmonary evaluation on all pts with skeletal muscle weakness.
■ Pts w/ signs of congestive heart failure should have a full cardiac workup.

PREOP EVALUATION
N/A

OPERATIVE PREPARATION
N/A

ANESTHESIA
■ Consider regional anesthesia to avoid the use of muscle relaxants.
■ General anesthesia

➤ Pts w/ Duchenne's muscular dystrophy are at higher risk of malignant hyperthermia, so avoid using triggering anesthetics.

➤ Smooth muscle involvement may result in hypomotility of the intestinal tract & delayed gastric emptying, so take precautions to prevent aspiration.

➤ There have been numerous reports of cardiac arrest w/ induction, so monitor cardiac function carefully.

➤ Monitoring is aimed at early detection of malignant hyperthermia & congestive heart failure.

➤ Because of possible prolonged paralysis, avoid or limit use of neuromuscular blocking agents.

➤ Marked respiratory & circulatory depression may be seen with the use of volatile anesthetics in pts w/ advanced disease.

➤ Pts w/ FVC <30% of predicted are at greatest risk of requiring postop ventilation.

WAKE UP & EMERGENCE
N/A

ICU AND PACU

■ Because of the potential for postop complications, observe pts overnight if more than a very minor procedure is performed.

■ Vigorous postop respiratory therapy can be helpful.

MYASTHENIA GRAVIS

KARL WILLMANN, MD AND D. B. COURSIN, MD

SCREENING AND EVALUATION

■ Duration & severity of symptoms, including bulbar dysfunction & respiratory dysfunction

- Evaluate pts w/ dyspnea or orthopnea for anterior mediastinal mass, including chest x-ray (CT), flow loop diagrams.
- PFTs
- Discuss w/ pt possibility of postop intubation.
  - ➤ Risks for prolonged intubation
    - Duration of disease >6 yrs
    - History of other chronic lung disease
    - Pyridostigmine (Mestinon) dose >750 mg/day
    - Preop vital capacity <2.9 L
- Discussion of postoperative analgesia (epidural, PCA, NSAID, etc.)
- Meds & doses, including steroids, immunosuppressive agents, including cyclosporine, azathioprine & mycophenolate, anticholinesterases, recent plasmapheresis or immunoglobulin
- Labs: CBC, platelets, electrolytes, BUN, CR, LFTs
- Thorough history of pt's symptoms & course of disease, looking for evidence of myasthenic or cholinergic crisis
- Myasthenic crisis, increased weakness & symptoms, is caused by too little acetylcholine & requires a higher dose of anticholinesterase.
- Cholinergic crisis is heralded by increasing weakness & cholinergic symptoms because of too much acetylcholine at the NMJ.
- Often it is hard to distinguish btwn the two entities; they can be delineated by giving a small dose of anticholinesterase (10 mg edrophonium); if the pt improves, myasthenic crisis is most likely.
- Neurology consult
- Optimize meds.
- MG symptoms should be at baseline.
- Evaluate pt for possible respiratory infections, which should be resolved before surgery.
- Pt may require plasmapheresis or immunoglobin to improve symptoms; arrange prior to surgery.

PREOPERATIVE PREPARATION

■ For pts w/ bulbar dysfunction, pretreat w/ metoclopramide, H2 blockers or proton pump inhibitor and/or non-particulate antacids.

■ Avoid or minimize use of narcotics for preop anxiolysis; they can depress respiratory function in pts w/ compromised status in unmonitored situations.

■ Pts on steroids may require stress-dose steroids.

■ May continue anticholinergic meds on day of surgery, especially pts who are dependent & awake w/ severe symptoms. Pts w/ more mild disease may skip the AM dose of anticholinergics if case is early in the morning.

■ MicroMedex states there is a 1:30 ratio IV to oral conversion of pyridostigmine (Mestinon).

OPERATIVE PREPARATION
N/A

ANESTHESIA

■ Induction

  ➤ If concern about large anterior mediastinal mass w/ large airway & vascular compression when pt supine, an awake fiberoptic intubation would be prudent.

  ➤ Pts w/ significant respiratory function or pts undergoing large abdominal or thoracic cases should have an arterial line.

  ➤ Rapid sequence induction w/ cricothyroid pressure for pts w/ bulbar dysfunction, understanding the altered pharmacology of both nondepolarizing & depolarizing muscle relaxants

  ➤ Intubation of the trachea w/ no muscle relaxation is optimal.

  ➤ MG pts are very sensitive to nondepolarizing agents, usually requiring only 10% of the normal dose, if needed.

➤ Pts are usually resistant to depolarizing agents & require 2–3 times the normal dose.

➤ Pts will have prolonged effect of depolarizing agents if they are treated w/ anticholinergic agents (inhibit pseudocholinesterase).

➤ Avoid long-acting muscle relaxants.

➤ Volatile agents have muscle-relaxing properties that are exaggerated in pts w/ MG & may be sufficient to provide the desired level of muscular relaxation.

■ Maintenance

➤ Regional anesthesia is acceptable, but techniques that block accessory muscles & rib cage muscles will increase respiratory function in pts w/ already decreased respiratory reserve.

WAKE UP AND EMERGENCE

■ Extubation criteria must be met:

➤ Pt must be fully awake w/ complete reversal of muscular blockade. Evaluate for cholinergic excess vs. muscular weakness.

➤ VC > 15 mL/kg

➤ A-a gradient O_2 > 350 mm Hg on 100% FIO_2

➤ $PaCO_2$ < 50 mm Hg

➤ Negative inspiratory force > -20 cm H_2O

➤ Stable cardiac status

➤ Warm

ICU OR PACU

■ Prolonged intubation & ventilation may be required.

■ Neurology consult

■ Continue steroids & anticholinesterases during the early postop period (if residual bulbar symptoms, pt may need gastric tube for medication administration).

■ Possible plasmapheresis & immunoglobin therapy to improve strength

NEUROLEPTIC MALIGNANT SYNDROME

HUGH R. PLAYFORD, MD

SCREENING AND EVALUATION
- Acute
  - Assess & optimize intravascular volume & hemodynamics.
  - Careful assessment of respiratory function, including ABGs
  - Assess serum potassium & indices of renal function.
  - Assess neurologic status.
- Chronic
  - Usually little changed from normal

PREOPERATIVE PREPARATION
- If possible, defer operative procedure until acute NMS has resolved.
- Avoid neuroleptic drugs (including metoclopramide).

OPERATIVE PREPARATION
- Avoid neuroleptic drugs (including metoclopramide).
- Acute
  - Use care w/ positioning if significant muscular rigidity

ANESTHESIA
- Avoid neuroleptic drugs (including metoclopramide).

WAKE UP AND EMERGENCE
N/A

ICU OR PACU
N/A

OBSTETRIC PATIENT HAVING INTERCURRENT SURGERY

JONATHAN T. KETZLER, MD

SCREENING AND EVALUATION

- If not emergent, consider delaying until second trimester.
  - ➤ Delaying to second trimester decreases the incidence of teratogenicity & spontaneous miscarriage.
  - ➤ Risk of preterm labor is lower in second trimester than it is in third trimester.
- Discuss w/ pt risks & benefits of anesthesia to fetus & pregnancy.
- Educate pt about signs & symptoms of preterm labor.

PREOPERATIVE PREPARATION

- Pain & anxiety elevate maternal catecholamine levels & may decrease uterine blood flow, so premedicate accordingly.
- Aspiration prophylaxis w/ H2-receptor antagonist, metoclopramide or antacid

OPERATIVE PREPARATION

- Discuss need for tocolysis w/ obstetrician.
  - ➤ Indomethacin & magnesium sulfate are most commonly used tocolytics.
  - ➤ Magnesium sulfate may potentiate muscle relaxants & make hypovolemic shock more refractory.

ANESTHESIA

- Avoid maternal hypoxemia & hypotension.
- Maintenance of uterine perfusion & maternal oxygenation to preserve fetal oxygenation are most important aspects. Left lateral tilt if possible to avoid aortocaval compression.
- Be cognizant of anesthetic effects on maternal cardiac output, oxygen delivery & uterine blood flow.

- Pregnancy outcome is not affected by type of anesthetic, type of surgery, length of anesthetic or surgical blood loss.
- Monitoring
  - BP
  - Pulse oximetry
  - End-tidal capnography
  - Temperature
  - After 24 wks gestation, intermittent or continuous fetal monitoring if it will not interfere w/ the surgical procedure
    - Loss of beat-to-beat variability is normal w/ anesthetics, but not decelerations.
    - Decelerations may indicate need to increase maternal oxygenation, raise BP, increase uterine displacement, change site of surgical retraction or begin tocolytics.
    - Fetal monitoring has not been shown to improve fetal outcome.
- General anesthesia
  - Very high likelihood of difficult airway
  - Full preoxygenation & denitrogenation
  - Rapid sequence induction w/ cricoid pressure
  - High concentration of oxygen
  - Slow reversal of muscle relaxants to avoid rapid increases in acetylcholine, which can induce uterine contraction
  - Keep MAC < 2.0 to prevent decreasing maternal cardiac output.
  - Propofol reduces oxytocin-induced contractions of uterine smooth muscle.
- Regional anesthesia
  - Minimizes drug exposure & changes in fetal heart rate
  - Prevent hypotension w/ adequate hydration & uterine displacement.
  - Treat hypotension aggressively w/ ephedrine.
  - Decrease neuraxial dose by about one third.
- Principles for anesthesia <24 wks gestation

➤ Delay surgery until second trimester if possible.
➤ Preop assessment by obstetrician
➤ Aspiration prophylaxis
➤ Monitor & maintain oxygenation, CO_2, BP & blood sugar.
➤ Use regional anesthesia when appropriate.
➤ Avoid high concentrations of nitrous oxide.
➤ Document fetal heart tones before & after anesthetic.
■ Principles for anesthesia >24 wks gestation
➤ Discuss use of tocolytics w/ obstetrician.
➤ Aspiration prophylaxis
➤ Maintain left uterine displacement at ALL times.
➤ Monitor & maintain oxygenation, CO_2, BP & blood sugar.
➤ Fetal monitoring intraoperatively when feasible
➤ Monitor for uterine contractions postop.
➤ Document fetal heart tones before & after anesthetic.

WAKE UP & EMERGENCE
N/A

ICU OR PACU
N/A

PARKINSON'S DISEASE

ROBERT N. SLADEN, MD

SCREENING AND EVALUATION
■ Severity of disease (very variable)
■ Signs of general debility
➤ Muscle wasting
➤ Poor nutritional status
■ Airway exam
➤ Limitation in mouth opening, neck mobility due to muscle rigidity

> Excessive secretions
- Relevant lab studies
  > Hct, CBC
  > Electrolytes (total CO_2 if ABG impracticable)
  > Blood sugar
  > BUN, creatinine
  > LFTs
  > ECG, chest x-ray

PREOPERATIVE PREPARATION
- Neurology consult
  > Severe disease
  > Recent change in status
  > Assist w/ drug optimization
- Anticipate dehydration (severe disease)
  > Establish venous access & provide judicious rehydration
- Anticipate difficult airway
  > Discuss w/ pt possible awake tracheal intubation.
  > Prepare difficult airway cart.

OPERATIVE PREPARATION
- Aspiration prophylaxis (anticipate difficult tracheal intubation)
  > Anticholinergic agent (glycopyrrolate preferred)
  > H_2 blocker (famotidine preferred)
  > Metoclopramide
  > Sodium bicitrate
- Anticipate difficult access
  > Peripheral IV, arterial line, IJ difficult w/ severe rigidity
- Careful positioning
  > Rigidity
  > Support & protect all affected joints w/ soft material.
  > Severe rigidity may render normal positioning impossible.
- Use active warming devices to prevent hypothermia
  > Forced-air convection blanket

ANESTHESIA

- Regional anesthesia
  - ➤ May be impossible in presence of severe rigidity
  - ➤ Anticipate hypotension (chronic dopaminergic vasodilation)
- General anesthesia
  - ➤ Anticipate difficult airway
  - ➤ Anticipate aspiration (excessive secretions)
  - ➤ Anticipate hyperreactive airways (excessive secretions)
  - ➤ Anticipate hypotension (chronic dopaminergic vasodilation)

WAKE UP AND EMERGENCE

- Careful planning for anesthetic emergence
  - ➤ If tracheal intubation was difficult, do not extubate until completely awake.
  - ➤ If in doubt, plan transient postop ventilation until airway protection is ensured.
- Potential complications on emergence
  - ➤ Vomiting, aspiration
  - ➤ Airway obstruction
  - ➤ Respiratory depression
  - ➤ Acute respiratory failure

ICU AND PACU

- Consider short period of postop mechanical ventilation (see above).
- Anticipate postop complications
  - ➤ Airway obstruction
  - ➤ Acute respiratory failure
  - ➤ Sepsis, wound dehiscence
  - ➤ Anemia
- Postop meds
  - ➤ Defer antiplatelet agents until no further risk of bleeding.

➤ Provide GI prophylaxis (H_2 blocker, proton pump inhibitor).

➤ Resume preop meds as soon as possible.

PATIENT WITH A TRANSPLANT

ARTHUR ATCHABAHIAN, MD

SCREENING AND EVALUATION

- 12-lead EKG
- Chest x-ray
- CBC, electrolytes, BUN, creatinine, glucose & liver function tests

Heart Tx

- Reason for Tx: CAD, dilated CM, viral myocarditis
- Evaluate cardiac function clinically (exercise tolerance, hypotension, JVD, pedal edema, signs of pulmonary edema on chest auscultation, gallop).
- Obtain consult from cardiologist regarding function of the transplant, coronary artery disease, current immunosuppressive therapy & history of rejection.
- Consider obtaining echocardiogram & noninvasive stress test if information not available.

Renal Tx

- Reason for Tx: diabetes mellitus, vasculitis, glomerulonephritis, uncontrolled hypertension, obstruction
- Evaluate renal function clinically (urine output & density) & biologically (BUN, creatinine, creatinine clearance if needed).
- Obtain consult from nephrologist regarding renal function & evolution, current immunosuppressive therapy & history of rejection.

Liver Tx

- Reason for transplant: cirrhosis w/ or w/out potential for recurrence, biliary malformation, acute hepatic failure
- Evaluate liver function clinically (ascites, encephalopathy, jaundice) & biologically (PT, serum bilirubin, serum lactate).
- Obtain consult from hepatologist regarding liver function, current immunosuppressive therapy & history of rejection.

Lung Tx

- Reason for Tx: cystic fibrosis, end-stage emphysema, alpha-1 antitrypsin deficiency, primary pulmonary hypertension
- Assess pulmonary function clinically (exercise tolerance, auscultation, cyanosis, pulse oximetry) & biologically (ABG, or total CO_2 on electrolyte panel).
- Obtain consult from pulmonologist regarding pulmonary function, current immunosuppressive therapy & history of rejection.

PREOPERATIVE PREPARATION

- Take all immunosuppressive meds on the morning of surgery.

OPERATIVE PREPARATION

- Strict aseptic technique because of susceptibility to infection
- Consider rapid sequence intubation if renal or hepatic Tx.
- Consider stress-dose steroids unless very low-dose steroid maintenance & minor surgery.
- Careful positioning
  - ➤ Fragile skin because of steroid treatment, renal or hepatic failure
  - ➤ Ascites

ANESTHESIA

Heart Tx

- Avoid right internal jugular central venous access, as this is the site used to perform myocardial biopsies.

- Maintain adequate preload; avoid sudden vasodilation.
- Treat hypotension by fluid administration & direct-acting agents such as phenylephrine & norepinephrine.
- Risk of myocardial ischemia if significant coronary artery disease

Renal Tx

- Maintain adequate fluid status to preserve renal perfusion.
- Closely monitor urine output; treat aggressively any oliguria.
- Avoid nephrotoxic meds (eg, radiologic contrast dye, aminoglycosides, vancomycin, diuretics).
- Theoretical risk of nephrotoxicity w/ enflurane & sevoflurane

Liver Tx

- Avoid hypotension & hepatotoxic meds (halothane).
- Succinylcholine effect can be prolonged (decreased pseudocholinesterase).
- If poor graft function, considerations for hepatic insufficiency apply
  - ➤ Decreased elimination of meds dependent on hepatic function
  - ➤ Hypoalbuminemia w/ decreased protein binding
  - ➤ Propensity to hypoglycemia
  - ➤ Coagulopathy, thrombocytopenia
  - ➤ Esophageal varices: discuss need for gastric tube and/or TEE

Lung Tx

- If poor graft function or single-lung transplant, possible need for postop ventilation

WAKE UP AND EMERGENCE

- Delayed awakening or recovery from neuromuscular blockade because of decreased elimination of drugs or metabolites
- Extubate when fully awake.

ICU OR PACU

Infections in the transplant recipient

- First month: nosocomial infections due to the same organisms (bacteria & fungi) as in immunocompetent surgical pts
- 1–6 months: viral & opportunistic infections (eg, *Pneumocystis carinii*)
- After 6 months: pts on high-dose immunosuppressants are exposed to opportunistic infections
  - ➤ *Listeria monocytogenes* (meningitis)
  - ➤ *Pneumocystis carinii* (pneumonia)
  - ➤ *Cryptococcus neoformans* (encephalitis)
  - ➤ Aspergillus, Candida (pneumonia or disseminated disease)
  - ➤ CMV (hepatitis, pneumonitis, enterocolitis & glomerulonephritis)
- Blunted signs of infection; therefore, consider periodic routine cultures
- Meticulous attention to drug interactions (eg, cyclosporine absorption decreased by sucralfate, allopurinol in combination w/ azathioprine can trigger severe leukopenia)
- GI prophylaxis for pts on steroids, esp. if other risk factors (eg, mechanical ventilation, coagulation disorder)
- Continue immunosuppressive treatment.
- Risk of critical illness myopathy in pts necessitating prolonged neuromuscular blockade & receiving steroids

---

PHEOCHROMOCYTOMA

GIUDITTA ANGELINI, MD

SCREENING AND EVALUATION

- The following are serum screening tests for pheochromocytoma:
  - ➤ 2,000 pg/mL plasma catecholamines

- ➤ >1,200 mcg urine catecholamines
- ➤ >100 mcg urine norepinephrine
- ➤ >1 mcg urine epinephrine
- ➤ >2.5 mg urine metanephrines
- ➤ >10 mg urine vanillylmandelic acid
- ➤ Not suppressed by clonidine
- ➤ Metanephrines most sensitive
- ■ MRI scan most helpful for extra-adrenal locations & pregnant pts
- ■ CT w/ I-131-labeled metaiodobenzyl guanidine extremely accurate
- ■ Arteriography can stimulate catecholamine release & should be used w/ extreme care.

PREOPERATIVE PREPARATION
- ■ Preop optimization w/ alpha blockers & intravascular volume expansion has reduced perioperative mortality from 45% to 0–3%.
- ■ Alpha blockers
  - ➤ Phenoxybenzamine orally for up to 10–14 days before surgery
  - ➤ Commence at 10–40 mg BID, but many need 80–200 mg/day.
  - ➤ Increase dose to control BP & paroxysms.
  - ➤ Irreversible binding of alpha receptors (presynaptic alpha-2 & postsynaptic alpha-1)
  - ➤ Long-acting (24–48 hrs)
  - ➤ Side effects: orthostatic hypotension, reflex tachycardia
  - ➤ Prazosin 2–5 mg BID orally before surgery
  - ➤ Competitive postsynaptic alpha-1 blocker
  - ➤ May be used alone or in addition to phenoxybenzamine for hemodynamic stability
  - ➤ Continue preoperative alpha blockers up to day of surgery.
  - ➤ Phentolamine often used intraoperatively

- Beta blockers
  - Used if tachycardia persists or arrhythmia develops w/ alpha blocker therapy
  - Use only after alpha blockade has been initiated (to avoid unopposed alpha agonism).
- Preoperative hypertensive crises
  - Managed w/ additional phentolamine, nitroprusside or fenoldopam
- Alpha-methyl tyrosine (inhibits tyrosine hydroxylase) may be used if surgery contraindicated or in the presence of metastatic disease.
  - Used in combination w/ alpha blockade
- Magnesium
- ACE inhibitors
- Calcium channel blockers
- Preop hydration crucial to allow intravascular volume expansion as the alpha blockade is introduced

OPERATIVE PREPARATION
- Avoid:
  - Droperidol (due to inhibition of catecholamine reuptake)
  - Atropine (exacerbates chronotropic effects of epinephrine)
  - Morphine, curare, atracurium (associated w/ histamine release)
  - Pancuronium, ketamine, ephedrine (indirectly stimulate catecholamine)
  - Halothane (myocardial irritability in the presence of high levels of catecholamines)
- Monitoring
  - V5 lead ECG, temperature, pulse oximetry, $ETCO_2$, arterial line, central line, urine catheter, PA catheter if myocardial dysfunction severe

ANESTHESIA

- Anesthetic
  - Most agents not listed above to avoid can be used.
  - Halothane may be avoided due to sensitization of myocardium to catecholamines.
  - Desflurane has been shown to be safe despite increase in sympathetic stimulation.
  - Regional anesthesia can be used but will likely not control episodic hypertension.
- Controlling catecholamine release
  - Nitroprusside 1–8 mcg/kg/min IV
  - Phentolamine 1–5 mg IV q5min or 1 mg/min continuous infusion
  - Labetalol 10–20 mg IV q10min to max 200 mg
  - Esmolol 10–20 mg IV q10min or 50–300 mcg/kg/min continuous
  - Hydralazine 10 mg IV q30min to max 40 mg
  - Magnesium sulfate 2 g IV up to 6 g w/out renal failure
- Hemodynamics after tumor removal
  - Hypotension common
  - Fluid hydration
  - Norepinephrine infusion may be required.
- Pregnancy
  - Magnesium particularly helpful in this group

WAKE UP & EMERGENCE

N/A

ICU OR PACU

- Increased sensitivity to narcotics after tumor removal
- Hypoglycemia is possible & should be monitored.
- Catecholamine levels do not decrease for several days after surgery.
- If hypertension continues, there may be residual pheochromocytoma.

PLATELET DISORDERS

KARL WILLMANN, MD

SCREENING AND EVALUATION

- Hematology consult is necessary. Discontinue drugs & therapies that have a negative impact on platelet count & function.
- Coagulation studies, including PTT, PT, fibrinogen, platelet count & thromboelastogram

PREOPERATIVE PREPARATION

- Have platelets available if appropriate for treatment.
- If anticoagulation needed in the presence of HIT, use direct thrombin inhibitor (eg, agatroban). Avoid all heparin preparations.
- In the presence of uremia-induced platelet dysfunction, consider DDAVP (0.3 mcg/kg IV) to improve platelet function.

OPERATIVE PREPARATION

N/A

ANESTHESIA

- Induction
  - ➤ Gentle laryngoscopy to avoid trauma & bleeding
  - ➤ Avoid nasal intubation.
- Maintenance
  - ➤ Regional anesthesia is relatively contraindicated in pts w/ bleeding diathesis.
  - ➤ Minimize/avoid hypothermia (increases sequestration).

WAKE UP AND EMERGENCE

- Avoid coughing & bucking on endotracheal tube, leading to bleeding.

ICU OR PACU

■ Continued monitoring of coagulation status; prompt treatment of platelet-related bleeding

■ Rewarm to normothermia to aid platelet function.

POLYCYTHEMIA

KARL WILLMANN, MD, AND DOUGLAS B. COURSIN, MD

SCREENING AND EVALUATION

■ Hct, Hgb, platelets, LFTs

PREOPERATIVE PREPARATION

■ Control Hct for all elective surgery. Pts usually have been undergoing phlebotomy to keep Hct values near normal. This should be continued. Hct near 46% is considered adequate.

■ Have platelets available if bleeding is encountered.

OPERATIVE PREPARATION

■ Take steps to reduce deep venous thrombosis during surgery, such as applying sequential compression stockings or appropriate anticoagulant prophylaxis.

ANESTHESIA

■ No specific concerns

WAKE UP AND EMERGENCE

■ No specific concerns

ICU OR PACU

■ No specific concerns other than the possibility of thrombosis & bleeding issues

PSYCHIATRIC DISORDERS

JONATHAN T. KETZLER, MD

SCREENING AND EVALUATION

- Depression
  - ➤ Investigate use of OTC meds such as St. John's wort.
  - ➤ Tricyclic antidepressants
    - Usually continued through perioperative period
  - ➤ MAOIs
    - In the past were discontinued 2 wks before surgery to allow regeneration of enzymes irreversibly inhibited by MAO inhibitors
    - But because patients on MAOIs usually have severe or refractory depression, continuing them through the perioperative period may be warranted on an individualized basis; this is still controversial.
    - If MAOIs are continued, keep drug/drug interactions in mind.
- Mania
  - ➤ Lithium
    - Greatest concern is perioperative toxicity.
    - Check serum lithium levels & electrolytes preoperatively.
      - Low serum sodium decreases renal excretion of lithium & can lead to toxicity.
      - There is no evidence that sodium loading is beneficial.
- Schizophrenia
  - ➤ Pts well controlled on meds usually pose few problems.
  - ➤ Continue meds through the perioperative period.

PREOP PREPARATION

N/A

OPERATIVE PREPARATION

N/A

ANESTHESIA

■ Depression

➤ Electroconvulsive therapy is being used more often for severe or refractory depression, primarily due to the safety added with general anesthesia.

- Tricyclic antidepressants
  - May increase anesthetic requirements secondary to enhanced brain catecholamine activity
  - Centrally acting anticholinergic agents may be potentiated, leading to postop confusion & delirium.
  - Response to both indirect-acting vasopressors & sympathomimetic agents may be enhanced.
    - Use caution when administering drugs such as pancuronium, ketamine, meperidine & epinephrine containing local anesthetics.
  - Chronic use of tricyclic antidepressants may deplete cardiac catecholamines, potentiating the myocardial depressant effect of anesthetics.
  - In the face of hypotension, use small doses of direct-acting vasopressors.
- MAOIs
  - Phenelzine may decrease levels of plasma cholinesterase, prolonging the duration of succinylcholine.
  - Use of meperidine in pts on MAOIs may result in hyperthermia & seizures.
  - MAOIs may exaggerate response to indirect-acting vasopressors & sympathomimetics.
    - Use caution when administering drugs such as pancuronium, ketamine, meperidine & epinephrine containing local anesthetics.

- In the face of hypotension, use small doses of direct-acting vasopressors.
- Mania
  - Lithium
    - Lithium toxicity may cause confusion, sedation, muscle weakness, tremor & slurred speech.
    - Higher concentrations may cause widening of the QRS complex, atrioventricular block, hypotension & seizures.
    - Fluid restriction & overdiuresis may lead to lithium toxicity.
    - Lithium may decrease minimum alveolar concentration.
    - Lithium may prolong duration of neuromuscular blocking agents.
- Schizophrenia
  - Well-medicated pts may require less anesthetic.
  - Antipsychotics may reduce the seizure threshold.

WAKE UP & EMERGENCE
N/A

ICU OR PACU
N/A

RESTRICTIVE LUNG DISEASE

HUGH R. PLAYFORD, MBBS

SCREENING AND EVALUATION
- Assess for severity of disease & any reversible components (esp. infection).
- Aside from the history & exam, consider chest x-ray, PFTs, ABGs, sputum culture & sensitivity.
- Identify & eradicate acute bacterial infection w/ antibiotics & physical therapy.

- Optimize nutritional state for good muscular strength w/out overfeeding-induced nutrition.
- Cease smoking.
- Most pts should have pneumococcal vaccine & yearly influenza vaccines.
- Assess pt for chronic steroid usage (will need perioperative coverage).
- Treat any cardiac dysfunction.
- Train pt in postop respiratory therapy techniques.

PREOPERATIVE PREPARATION

- Eradicate any pulmonary infection.
- Optimize pulmonary therapy.
- Consider physical therapy & nutrition.
- Pts are at increased risk of developing acute respiratory failure during postop period.
- Plan intraoperative technique (regional, general, combined) & postop analgesic regimen to have minimal pulmonary detriment.

OPERATIVE PREPARATION

- Antibiotics if needed
- Influenza vaccination
- Diuresis for cor pulmonale & right heart failure
- Supplemental oxygen titrated to pt's needs
- Physical training programs

ANESTHESIA

- Regional anesthesia
  - ➤ Potentially avoids respiratory depressant effects of sedative drugs
  - ➤ Avoid regional techniques that provide sensory anesthesia above T6 to T10 (may decrease expiratory reserve volume & impair effectiveness to cough & clear secretions).

- General anesthesia
  - Volatile anesthesia allows humidification, anesthesia delivery w/ a relatively rapid onset & offset, blunting of airway reflexes & reflex bronchospasm, & volatile-induced bronchodilatation.
  - Volatile anesthesia also attenuates regional hypoxic pulmonary vasoconstriction, leading to increased right-to-left intrapulmonary shunting.
  - Nitrous oxide techniques limit the FiO2 that can be delivered.
  - Opioids may lead to prolonged respiratory depression; use judiciously.
  - Humidification is used to prevent drying of secretions in the airways.
- If intubation is necessary, goals are:
  - Adequate arterial oxygenation
  - Avoiding ventilator-induced lung injury (barotrauma, volutrauma)
    - Ventilate w/ a similar technique to protective lung ventilation for pts w/ ARDS.
    - Tidal volumes of 6–7 mL/kg, respiratory rate of 20–30 breaths/min to achieve airway plateau pressures of <35 cm H_2O
    - May need modification if hypercapnia of concern (depresses myocardial function, increases intracranial pressure)

WAKE UP AND EMERGENCE

- Principles are to have the pt well analgesed w/ good effective cough & deep inspiration w/out any residual respiratory depression.
- Extubation
  - Ideally, extubate at the end of the surgical procedure (depends on procedure & duration of anesthesia).

➤ Tracheal tube increases airway resistance & risk of reflex bronchoconstriction, limits the pt's ability to clear secretions effectively & increases the risk of iatrogenic infection.

■ Analgesia
  ➤ Regional techniques using local anesthesia and/or neuraxial opioids may be able to avoid significant respiratory depression.
  ➤ Neuraxial local anesthesia may lead to postural hypotension & interfere w/ postop ambulation & sputum clearance & incentive spirometry.
  ➤ Pt-controlled analgesia w/ systemic opioids may also minimize the risk of significant respiratory depression.
  ➤ With any route of opioid, however, potent respiratory depression may develop; epidural opioids may depress ventilation up to 12 hrs after administration.
  ➤ Consider other nonrespiratory depressing analgesics as adjunctive agents (acetaminophen, alpha-2 agonists such as clonidine and dexmedetomidine, NSAIDs).

■ Chest physical therapy & incentive spirometry

ICU OR PACU
■ Continued intubation & ventilation in the postop period may be necessary in pts after major upper abdominal or thoracic surgery.
■ Discontinuation of ventilation is based on the pt's clinical condition (preexisting pulmonary impairment, surgical procedure, duration of anesthesia) as well as indices of respiratory function.
  ➤ The changes in pulmonary function that occur postop are primarily restrictive; these changes added to preexisting restrictive lung disease may be catastrophic in the individual pt.
  ➤ Proportional decreases in all lung volumes; no change in airway resistance

➤ FRC decreases from decreased abdominal excursion (eg, from abdominal operations), abnormal postop respiratory pattern (shallow, rapid breaths).

➤ Operative site is the most important factor.

➤ Non-laparoscopic upper abdominal operations decrease FRC by 40–50% > lower abdominal & thoracic operations decrease FRC by 30% > other operative sites decrease FRC by 15–20%.

RHEUMATOID ARTHRITIS

ROBERT N. SLADEN, MD

SCREENING AND EVALUATION

■ Signs of general debility

➤ Mild, moderate or severe (important impact on overall planning)

➤ Fixed deformities

➤ Major joint deformity (knees, hips, wrists)

➤ Poor nutritional status

■ Airway exam

➤ Jaw opening (temporomandibular joint)

➤ Neck mobility (atlantoaxial joint, odontoid process)

➤ Fixed flexion deformity of neck

■ Signs of steroid therapy

➤ Muscle wasting, poor skin turgor, ecchymoses

➤ Cushing's syndrome (includes hypertension, hyperglycemia)

■ Relevant lab studies

➤ Hct, CBC

➤ Electrolytes (total CO_2 if ABG impracticable)

➤ Blood sugar

➤ BUN, creatinine

➤ LFTs

➤ ECG, chest x-ray
➤ PFTs & ABGs (if restrictive lung disease suspected)

PREOPERATIVE PREPARATION
■ Discontinue aspirin & NSAIDs prior to major surgery
  ➤ Aspirin: 7 days prior to surgery
  ➤ NSAIDs: 24 hrs prior to surgery
  ➤ Evaluate risk-benefit of analgesia vs. increased bleeding risk.
■ Adrenal support for major surgery, stress
  ➤ Start hydrocortisone 100 mg IV q8h, taper over next 24–72 hrs.
■ Anticipate dehydration (severe disease)
  ➤ Establish venous access & provide judicious rehydration.
  ➤ Anticipate difficult airway
    • Discuss possible awake tracheal intubation w/ pt.
    • Prepare difficult airway cart.

OPERATIVE PREPARATION
■ Aspiration prophylaxis (anticipate difficult tracheal intubation)
  ➤ Anticholinergic agent (glycopyrrolate preferred)
  ➤ H_2 blocker (famotidine preferred)
  ➤ Metoclopramide
  ➤ Sodium bicitrate
■ Use universal & aseptic precautions throughout (steroid, immunosuppressive therapy).
■ Anticipate difficult access
  ➤ Peripheral IV, arterial line, IJ difficult w/ severe deformity
■ Careful positioning
  ➤ Fragile skin, easy bruising
  ➤ Support & protect all affected joints w/ soft material.
  ➤ Severe deformity may render normal positioning impossible.

- Use active warming devices to prevent hypothermia
  - Forced-air convection blanket

ANESTHESIA

- Regional anesthesia
  - Not precluded by aspirin, NSAIDs
  - May be impossible in presence of severe deformity
  - Difficult airway is not a sole indication for regional anesthesia.
  - May be faced w/ emergency intubation in total spinal
- General anesthesia
  - Anticipate difficult airway.
  - Notify surgeon to be present, tracheotomy backup.
- Anesthetic induction for difficult airway
  - Awake fiberoptic intubation preferred
  - If not tolerated, consider inhalation induction w/ spontaneous breathing, then attempt fiberoptic intubation.
  - If unsuccessful, place intubating LMA, then attempt tracheal intubation via LMA.
  - If unsuccessful, proceed w/ tracheotomy.
  - Restrictive lung disease
    - Avoid excessive tidal volumes.
    - May require rapid, shallow ventilation

WAKE UP AND EMERGENCE

- Careful planning for anesthetic emergence
  - If tracheal intubation was difficult, do not extubate until pt is completely awake.
  - If in doubt, plan transient postop ventilation until airway protection is ensured.
  - Consider dexmedetomidine infusion (0.2–0.4 mcg/kg/hr)
    - Provides endotracheal tube tolerance, analgesia & anxiolysis w/out respiratory depression
    - Allows careful assessment of airway & ability to meet extubation criteria

- Potential complications on emergence
  - ➤ Vomiting, aspiration
  - ➤ Airway obstruction
  - ➤ Respiratory depression
  - ➤ Acute respiratory failure

ICU AND PACU
- Consider short period of postop mechanical ventilation (see above).
  - ➤ Anticipate postop complications
    - Airway obstruction
    - Hyperglycemia, hypertension (Cushing's syndrome)
    - Acute respiratory failure
    - Sepsis, wound dehiscence
    - Anemia
- Postop meds
  - ➤ Defer antiplatelet agents until no further risk of bleeding.
  - ➤ Provide GI prophylaxis (H_2 blocker, proton pump inhibitor).
  - ➤ Steroid taper over 24–72 hrs to maintenance dose
  - ➤ Resume preop meds as soon as possible.

SCLERODERMA

ARTHUR ATCHABAHIAN, MD

SCREENING AND EVALUATION
- Evaluate potential for difficult intubation because of retraction of soft tissues around mouth & TMJ stiffness.
- BUN & creatinine to assess renal function
- PFTs to determine severity of restrictive disease
- EKG to assess dysrhythmias or conduction abnormalities
- Consider echocardiography for assessment of ventricular function, pericardial effusion & pulmonary artery pressures.

- PT (INR) to rule out coagulation disorder

PREOPERATIVE PREPARATION

- ACE inhibitors may improve renal insufficiency or slow progression.
- Broad-spectrum antibiotics & vitamin K to treat coagulation disorder due to malabsorption & bacterial overgrowth

OPERATIVE PREPARATION

- Consider anti-H_2 1–2 hrs preop.
- Administer non-particulate antacid (Bicitra) just before entering OR.
- Keep operating temperature high to prevent vasoconstriction.

ANESTHESIA

- Difficult IV access because of skin thickening
  - ➤ Central venous catheterization might be needed.
- Consider awake fiberoptic intubation, possibly nasal, if mouth opening is very limited.
- Oral or nasal telangiectasias
  - ➤ Insert ETT & NGT w/ care.
- Vasoconstriction may interfere w/ pulse oximetry & NIBP monitoring.
  - ➤ Consider digital block to improve blood flow.
  - ➤ Use Doppler for BP.
  - ➤ Arterial catheterization can induce severe spasm.
- Beta blockers & ergot alkaloids can precipitate severe Raynaud's phenomenon.
  - ➤ Weigh benefit & risks.
- Contracted intravascular compartment w/ severe hypotension on induction
- Pulmonary fibrosis can make ventilation difficult w/ high airway pressures.
  - ➤ Do not use spontaneous ventilation w/ general anesthesia.
- Avoid nitrous oxide if possible because of its pulmonary vasoconstrictive effect.

- Limit opioid use because of effect on gut motility & respirations.
- Protect eyes.
- Consider renal function when choosing anesthetic agents.
- Prolonged effects of local anesthetics have been described.
  - ➤ Regional anesthesia may be difficult because of skin & joint abnormalities.
- Warm IV fluids & use warming blanket to prevent vasoconstriction.

WAKEUP AND EMERGENCE
- Possible delayed emergence because of higher sensitivity to opioids
- Postop ventilation may be indicated.

ICU OR PACU
- Consider postop ventilation because of pulmonary fibrosis.
- Use decreased doses of opioids because of effect on gut motility & higher sensitivity.
- Prevent or treat hypothermia.
- Monitoring issues as above due to vasoconstriction
- Skin ulcerates easily, heals poorly & is at higher risk for infection because of poor blood flow.
- Elevate head of bed by 30 degrees to prevent reflux & aspiration.
- Carefully follow renal function.

SICKLE CELL DISEASE

ARTHUR ATCHABAHIAN, MD

SCREENING AND EVALUATION
- Obtain CBC to assess anemia.
- Evaluate renal function (BUN, creatinine).
- Evaluate hepatic function (PT, bilirubin).

- Consider echocardiogram to evaluate ventricular function.
- Chest x-ray & ABGs to assess pulmonary involvement

PREOPERATIVE PREPARATION
- Consider partial exchange transfusion
  - ➤ Remove 15 mL/kg whole blood.
  - ➤ Replace w/ 20 mL/kg RBCs to bring HbA to at least 40%.
  - ➤ Depends on severity of anemia & type of surgery
  - ➤ Risks of transfusion include bone marrow depression & hyperviscosity.
- Admit 1 day preop to ensure adequate IV hydration.

OPERATIVE PREPARATION
- Warm up operating room.
- Place warming blanket on pt as soon as possible.
- Warm all IV fluid.

ANESTHESIA
- CPB poses a special threat:
  - ➤ Consider using high blood flow & normothermia.
- Meticulous attention to avoiding hypothermia
  - ➤ Warm up room.
  - ➤ Use low fresh gas flows & heat/moisture exchanger.
  - ➤ Warm IV fluids
  - ➤ Use warming blanket on pt.
- Meticulous attention to avoiding hypoxemia, acidosis & low peripheral blood flow
  - ➤ Maintain hemodynamic stability.
  - ➤ Maintain adequate hydration.
  - ➤ Pay special attention to positioning.
  - ➤ Consider using mixed venous oxygen saturation monitoring to guide therapy.
- Administration of bicarbonate is controversial & should not be routine.
- Do not use orthopedic tourniquet.

- Use prudence w/ succinylcholine (reports of decreased plasma cholinesterase activity).
- Central neuraxial blockade
  - Compensatory vasoconstriction in nonblocked areas w/ possible sickling
  - Maintains pulmonary function
  - Decreases blood loss & incidence of thromboembolic events

WAKE UP AND EMERGENCE
- Treat pain aggressively.
- Meticulously prevent or treat hypoxemia & acidosis.

ICU OR PACU
- Treat pain aggressively w/ major analgesics.
- Chest physiotherapy to prevent pulmonary infections
- Early ambulation
- Administer supplemental oxygen for several days.
- Maintain intravascular fluid status & body temperature.

SPINAL CORD INJURY

HUGH R. PLAYFORD, MBBS, AND GEBHARD WAGENER, MD

SCREENING AND EVALUATION
- Neurologic
  - Document neurologic deficits.
- Cardiovascular
  - Acute injury associated w/ hypotension, bradycardia, hypovolemia related to other injuries
  - Chronic injury related to risk of mass reflex
- Respiratory
  - Poor respiratory reserve

> ➤ Pt may have a chronic respiratory acidosis related to chronic hypoventilation.
> ➤ Hypoxia & widened arterial-alveolar gradient related to pulmonary collapse/atelectasis
> ➤ Consider PFTs, ABGs, chest x-ray.
- Electrolytes
  > ➤ Hyponatremia, acutely
  > ➤ Hypercalcemia, chronically
- Hematologic
  > ➤ Acute injury: anemia usually related to other injuries
  > ➤ Chronic injury: coagulopathy related to exogenous anti-coagulants

PREOPERATIVE PREPARATION
- Premeds (narcotics, sedatives) need to be titrated carefully in a monitored setting (OR) because of the risk of hypoventilation.
- Use care w/ premeds in acute injury that may impair neurologic exam.
- Atropine may counteract the vagal effects of some agents used during anesthesia.
- If a regional technique is considered, a rigorous neurologic exam is needed to accurately define the neurologic deficit.

OPERATIVE PREPARATION
- Monitoring
  > ➤ Acute injury: Invasive hemodynamic monitoring may be needed, depending on the severity of the injury, other injuries & the invasiveness of the surgery. SSEP may be important for spinal stabilization & decompression procedures.
  > ➤ Chronic injury: Monitoring depends on the pt's state & the invasiveness of the surgery.
- Positioning & transportation
  > ➤ Pay careful attention to these in both acute & chronic injury.

➤ Acute injury: Position pt awake to avoid exacerbating spinal cord injury. Reverse Trendelenburg & similar positions may have significant adverse hemodynamic consequences.

➤ Chronic injury: Be aware of contractures, pressure points & existing pressure sores.

■ Fasting

➤ Acute injury: Consider to be a "full stomach" secondary to gastric atony, supine positioning, paralyzed abdominal muscles & gastric tube.

■ Attempt to have pt awake, able to be neurologically assessed, well analgesed & w/ minimal respiratory depression at conclusion of anesthesia.

ANESTHESIA

■ Succinylcholine is contraindicated in the presence of spinal cord injury.

➤ Hyperkalemic response is related to the extrajunctional cholinergic receptor proliferation of denervated muscle.

➤ Develops within 1 day & lasts up to 9 months after injury

➤ Degree of hyperkalemia is proportional to the amount of muscle involved (not the dose of succinylcholine).

■ Cricoid pressure must be applied cautiously (but effectively) in pts w/ unstable cervical & upper thoracic spinal cord injury.

■ Longitudinal neck stabilization is required throughout intubation.

■ Method of intubation

➤ Depends on pt's condition, degree of neurologic injury, preference & experience of anesthesiologist, & whether the injury is acute or chronic

■ Temperature regulation

➤ Lesions above T1 may interfere w/ thermoregulation; esp. in the presence of anesthesia, pt may become poikilothermic.

WAKE UP AND EMERGENCE

- Extubate when pt meets extubation criteria, is awake & interactive, is able to cough & has minimal pulmonary secretions.
- Careful monitoring of respiratory status
  - ➤ Pt will need intense physiotherapy to mobilize pulmonary secretions in the postop period.
- Careful neurologic assessment for operatively related neural deterioration

ICU OR PACU

- Respiratory support may need to be continued into the postop period.
- Avoid significant postop respiratory depression w/ residual anesthesia/sedation or analgesia.

STROKE

GEBHARD WAGENER, MD

SCREENING AND EVALUATION

Pts w/ stroke:

- Avoid elective surgery at least 6 wks after stroke.
- Autoregulation, CO_2 responsiveness & blood-brain barrier abnormalities may persist for wks.
- Cardiac evaluation recommended for high-risk surgery: potential for concomitant coronary artery disease
- Coagulation profile, platelet count: hypercoagulable?
- BUN/creatinine, hematocrit: dehydration?
- Creatinine: renal vascular disease
- Glucose: avoid hyperglycemia
- pH, pCO_2: maintain moderate hypocarbia

To prevent perioperative stroke:

- Evaluate risk factors
- If high risk, pt will require:

➤ Cardiac evaluation: stress test, echocardiogram
- Assess:
  - ➤ Baseline BP
  - ➤ Degree of carotid stenosis

PREOPERATIVE PREPARATION

Pts w/ stroke:
- Adequate hydration: start IV maintenance fluid when NPO
- Assess & document neurologic deficits.

OPERATIVE PREPARATION

N/A

ANESTHESIA

For carotid endarterectomy (CEA)
- No benefit of awake CEA vs. general anesthesia w/ EEG monitoring vs. SSEP vs. transcranial Doppler: stroke more likely embolic than ischemic
- General placement of shunt or measurement of stump pressure alone not beneficial
- Regional anesthesia:
  - ➤ Advantage: more sensitive, no specialized knowledge necessary
  - ➤ Disadvantage: higher cerebral metabolic rate in awake state, pt cooperation essential
- If EEG used:
  - ➤ Get reliable baseline EEG.
  - ➤ Maintain even levels of anesthesia to evaluate changes in EEG.
  - ➤ Maintain blood pressure 30–50% above baseline during clamping of the carotid artery.
  - ➤ Use short-acting anesthetics allowing rapid postop recovery.
- Experience of anesthesiologist & center should determine technique.

- Surgical manipulation of carotid sinus can cause bradycardia.

To prevent perioperative stroke:

- There is no evidence that regional anesthesia is beneficial in preventing perioperative stroke.
- Avoid manipulation of neck & extreme neck rotation/ flexion/extension w/ carotid disease.
- Set target and acceptable BP range; treat any BP outside the acceptable range.
- Maintain BP at least as high as baseline pressure in high-risk pts.
- Regional anesthesia may allow monitoring of mental status & detection of new strokes during surgery.

WAKE UP AND EMERGENCE

Pts w/ stroke:

After general anesthesia:

- Wake up may be delayed
- Previously restored neurologic deficits may reappear temporarily in the immediate postop period.

To prevent perioperative stroke:

- Avoid hypotension & severe hypertension during emergence.
- Hypertension may cause hemorrhagic conversion of an ischemic stroke.
  - ➤ If a new stroke is suspected:
    - Keep pt endotracheally intubated.
    - Elevate head 30 degrees to decrease intracranial pressure.
    - Increase BP to maintain CPP.
    - Obtain immediate head CT scan.
    - Consider early (<3 hrs after stroke) angiogram & angioplasty.

ICU OR PACU

Pts w/ stroke:

- Admit to ICU.

After CEA:
- ICU preferable
- Observe for 24 hrs.
- Likely require invasive BP monitoring & aggressive control
- Rule out myocardial infarction.

SUBACUTE BACTERIAL ENDOCARDITIS PROPHYLAXIS

JONATHAN T. KETZLER, MD

SCREENING & EVALUATION
N/A

PREOPERATIVE PREPARATION

Treatment Recommendations for Common Invasive Procedures

Dental procedures
- Endocarditis prophylaxis recommended
  - Dental extractions
  - Periodontal procedures
  - Dental implant placement & reimplantation of avulsed teeth
  - Root canal instrumentation
  - Prophylactic cleaning of teeth or implants where bleeding is anticipated
- Endocarditis prophylaxis not recommended
  - Restorative dentistry
  - Local anesthetic injections (non-intraligamentary)
  - Intracanal endodontic treatment; postplacement & buildup
  - Placement of rubber dams
  - Postop suture removal

➤ Placement of removal prosthodontic or orthodontic appliances
➤ Taking of oral impressions
➤ Fluoride treatments
➤ Taking of oral radiographs
➤ Orthodontic appliance adjustment
➤ Shedding of primary teeth

Oral, respiratory, esophageal, other procedures

■ Endocarditis prophylaxis recommended
➤ Tonsillectomy or adenoidectomy
➤ Surgical operations involving respiratory mucosa
➤ Rigid bronchoscopy
➤ Flexible bronchoscopy w/ biopsy
■ Endocarditis prophylaxis not recommended
➤ Endotracheal intubation
➤ Flexible bronchoscopy (w/out biopsy)
➤ Tympanostomy tube insertion/removal
➤ Transesophageal echocardiography
➤ Cardiac catheterization including device placement
➤ Skin biopsy

Gastrointestinal, genitourinary procedures

■ Endocarditis prophylaxis recommended
➤ Biliary tract surgery
➤ Surgical operations involving intestinal mucosa
➤ Cystoscopy
➤ Urethral dilation
■ Endocarditis prophylaxis not recommended
➤ GI endoscopy w/out biopsy
➤ Vaginal delivery
➤ Cesarean section
➤ Urinary catheterization w/out infection
➤ Circumcision

OPERATIVE PREPARATION

N/A

ANESTHESIA

N/A

WAKE UP & EMERGENCE

N/A

ICU OR PACU

N/A

SYSTEMIC LUPUS ERYTHEMATOSUS

ARTHUR ATCHABAHIAN, MD

SCREENING AND EVALUATION

- Assess renal function w/ BUN & creatinine; look for recent change.
- Hct, white cell & platelet count to rule out anemia, leukopenia & thrombocytopenia
- Chest x-ray & EKG; consider echocardiogram, depending on clinical presentation

PREOPERATIVE PREPARATION

- Continue all meds until day of surgery.

OPERATIVE PREPARATION

- Unremarkable

ANESTHESIA

- No increased risk of exacerbation, even w/ meds known to induce lupus
- Consider administering stress-dose steroids.
- Consider renal function in choice of anesthetic agents.

- No correlation between lab tests & risk of bleeding. Rely on clinical exam (bruising, petechiae) to assess risk of central neuraxial block.
- Possible difficult mask fit if prominent nasal & malar cutaneous lesions
- Rare reports of cricoarytenoid arthritis w/ narrowed airway
- Ventilation can be difficult if restrictive disease.
- Consider antibiotic prophylaxis for bacterial endocarditis.
- Consider DVT prophylaxis if prolonged procedure.

WAKE UP AND EMERGENCE

- Possible need for postop ventilation if severe restrictive disease

ICU OR PACU

- Monitor EKG for arrhythmias.
- DVT prophylaxis because of hypercoagulable tendency
- Follow renal function.
  - ➤ Acute renal failure possible following surgical stress
  - ➤ Adjust medication dosing for renal function.
- Monitor CBC for anemia.
- Follow-up platelet count

THALASSEMIA

ARTHUR ATCHABAHIAN, MD

SCREENING AND EVALUATION

- Diagnosis by electrophoresis of Hb
- Obtain CBC to assess anemia & platelet count.
- Obtain PT to rule out coagulation disorder.
- Obtain EKG to assess rhythm.
- Consider obtaining echocardiogram to evaluate ventricular function.

PREOPERATIVE PREPARATION
Transfuse to Hb of 9 g/dL.

OPERATIVE PREPARATION
Unremarkable

ANESTHESIA
- Deformity of the maxilla can render intubation difficult.
- Careful positioning because of bone fragility & deformities
- Discuss risks & benefits of regional anesthesia
  - Coagulopathy, thrombocytopenia
  - No airway instrumentation, no cardiac depression
  - Decreased blood loss & thromboembolic events
- Consider renal & hepatic function for anesthetic drug selection.
- Consider invasive monitoring if cardiac function is compromised.

WAKE UP AND EMERGENCE
Unremarkable

ICU OR PACU
Unremarkable

THYROID AND PARATHYROID DISEASE

GIUDITTA ANGELINI, MD

SCREENING AND EVALUATION
- Indications for thyroidectomy
  - Suspected malignancy
  - Obstructive symptoms
  - Retrosternal goiter
  - Hyperthyroidism unresponsive to medical mgt
  - Cosmetic reasons or patient anxiety

- Assess for abnormalities of thyroid function & symptoms of thyroid disease.
- Cardiorespiratory assessment mandatory in pts w/ hyper- or hypothyroidism
- Before surgery, obtain thyroid function tests, CBC, electrolytes, urea & calcium in pts w/ hyper- or hypothyroidism.
- Anticipate difficult airway:
  - ➤ Symptoms (dysphagia, positional dyspnea)
  - ➤ Lingual thyroid
  - ➤ ENT evaluation w/ indirect laryngoscopy: vocal cord assessment
  - ➤ Chest x-ray: tracheal compression & deviation
  - ➤ CT & MRI: associated abnormalities & ease of intubation (not routinely done)
  - ➤ Respiratory flow volume loops
    - • Fixed obstruction: impaired inspiration/expiration
    - • Variable intrathoracic obstruction: impaired expiration
    - • Variable extrathoracic obstruction: impaired inspiration
- Very large goiters
  - ➤ Usually not as problematic as retrosternal goiter
  - ➤ Potential difficult intubation; lifting goiter anteriorly helps
  - ➤ Prolonged surgical time, postop tracheomalacia
  - ➤ Blood loss related to thyroid resection (rarely done today)
- Retrosternal goiter
  - ➤ Superior vena cava syndrome w/ or w/out thrombosis
  - ➤ Cerebral hypoperfusion from arterial compression
  - ➤ Thyrocervical steal syndrome
  - ➤ Phrenic & recurrent laryngeal nerve palsies
  - ➤ Horner's syndrome
  - ➤ Pleural effusion, pericardial effusion, chylothorax
- Thyroid cancer
  - ➤ Increased risk of recurrent laryngeal n. damage

- ➤ Follicular cancer: lung & bone metastases release thyroxin
- ➤ Lymphoma & anaplastic thyroid cancer are treated w/ radiotherapy alone.
- ▪ Investigate for multiple endocrine neoplasia (MEN).
  - ➤ MEN 1
    - • Hyperparathyroidism, parathyroid tumors, pancreatic tumors, pituitary adenomas
  - ➤ MEN 2
    - • Medullary thyroid cancer, pheochromocytoma, hyperparathyroidism
    - • Positive genetic screen for proto-oncogene mutation for medullary thyroid cancer is an indication for prophylactic thyroidectomy.

PREOPERATIVE PREPARATION

- ▪ Reschedule elective surgery if pt is not clinically euthyroid.
- ▪ Consider stress-dose steroids in hypothyroid pts (high incidence of concomitant adrenocortical deficiency).
- ▪ Symptomatic hypercalcemia & hyperparathyroidism
  - ➤ Preop saline + diuresis (saliuresis)
  - ➤ Bisphosphonates

OPERATIVE PREPARATION
N/A

ANESTHESIA

- ▪ Anticipate postop nausea & vomiting; pain is less of an issue after thyroidectomy.
- ▪ Hypothyroidism
  - ➤ Very sensitive to anesthetics & sedatives
  - ➤ Depressed response to hypoxemia, hypercarbia
- ▪ Regional anesthesia for thyroidectomy & parathyroidectomy
  - ➤ Bilateral superficial & deep cervical blocks

➤ Complications: vertebral artery puncture, epidural subarachnoid spread, bilateral phrenic n. block

■ LMA
  ➤ Requires close cooperation btwn surgeon & anesthesiologist as surgical manipulation can result in laryngospasm
  ➤ Contraindicated in pts w/ tracheal narrowing or deviation
  ➤ Allows assessment of vocal cord movement w/ fiberoptic scope during stimulation of recurrent laryngeal nerve
  ➤ Intubating LMA is difficult in pts w/ large goiter because of tracheal deviation.

■ Anticipate difficult intubation:
  ➤ 6% of tracheal intubations for thyroid surgery are likely to be difficult.
  ➤ No abnormality specific to thyroid disease reliably predicts difficulty.
  ➤ Consider using a small, reinforced tube in all pts, esp. pts w/ any amount of tracheal compression.
  ➤ Have LMA, fiberoptic scope, transtracheal jet ventilation available.
  ➤ Tracheotomy with femoro-femoral bypass has been used in severe airway obstruction.

■ General anesthesia: method of choice for pts w/ exophthalmos requiring eye surgery

■ Thyroid storm
  ➤ Surgery, infection & trauma are all triggers.
  ➤ Supportive treatment: hydration, cooling & inotropes
  ➤ First-line treatment includes anti-thyroxine agents & beta blockers.
  ➤ Magnesium decreases incidence & severity of catecholamine-induced arrhythmias.
  ➤ Dantrolene (1 mg/kg) has been used successfully in pts mistaken for MH

■ Intraoperative evaluation for recurrent laryngeal nerve
  ➤ Use succinylcholine for intubation.

- ➤ Place ETT w/ integrated EMG electrodes at level of vocal cords.
- ➤ Spontaneous ventilation should resume by time of testing.
- ➤ Once recurrent laryngeal n. localized, stimulation w/ 0.1 mA is repeated w/ 0.05-mA increments until an evoked EMG is obtained.
- ■ Medullary & papillary thyroid cancer
  - ➤ Can spread to lymph nodes & may require block resection in the neck
- ■ Sternotomy: rarely required, even w/ retrosternal goiter
- ■ 10–20 seconds of sustained positive pressure before wound closure is helpful to ensure hemostasis.
- ■ Risks of parathyroid surgery
  - ➤ 0.5%: injury to recurrent laryngeal nerve
  - ➤ 0.5%: risk of damage to normal parathyroid glands
  - ➤ 1%: risk of failure to identify adenoma
  - ➤ Parathyroid cancer requires en bloc resection w/ regional lymph node metastases.

WAKE UP AND EMERGENCE

- ■ Extubation should be done w/ minimal coughing.
  - ➤ Consider deep extubation or lidocaine suppression.
  - ➤ Consider dexmedetomidine through emergence.
- ■ Vocal cord injury
  - ➤ Concern re recurrent laryngeal n:
    - • Inspect vocal cords w/ fiberoptic scope before extubation.
    - • Place LMA at the end of surgery while pt is spontaneously breathing.
  - ➤ Unilateral vocal cord paralysis
    - • Hoarseness, breathlessness, ineffective cough & aspiration
    - • Temporary (3–4%)
    - • Permanent (<1%)

- Due to ischemia, contusion, traction, entrapment, transection
- Intracordal injection, laryngeal reinnervation & surgical corrective procedures can be done for permanent unilateral paralysis.
➤ Bilateral vocal cord paralysis
  - Stridor at extubation
  - Pt should be reintubated.
  - Permanent: consider tracheostomy
■ Tracheomalacia
  ➤ Unlike deviation & compression of the trachea, which resolve immediately, tracheomalacia persists.
  ➤ Develops in 5% of pts w/ tracheal compression
  ➤ Suggested by absence of cuff leak at the end of procedure or less air in cuff to create a seal
  ➤ Pt will require tracheostomy & potentially some form of tracheal support.

ICU OR PACU
■ Monitor for respiratory obstruction:
  ➤ Myxedema: rarely, laryngeal edema in isolation w/out associated hematoma
  ➤ Indirect laryngoscopy can also be used postop if vocal cord dysfunction is suspected in the extubated pt.
  ➤ Cervical hematoma
    - Reoperation rate is 0.4% in 3,000 cases.
    - Can produce laryngeal or pharyngeal edema w/ potential for emergent & difficult intubation
■ Total thyroidectomy pts who were not on replacement should receive thyroxine.
■ Inadvertent parathyroidectomy
  ➤ May be removed in about 20% of total thyroidectomy cases
  ➤ Calcium evaluation & potential replacement may be necessary.
  ➤ Only about 3% remain permanently hypocalcemic

TRANSFUSION THERAPY

DOUGLAS B. COURSIN, MD, AND KARL WILLMANN, MD

SCREENING AND EVALUATION

- Type & screen or cross-match, usually based on type of surgery, likelihood of blood loss & underlying health & Hgb of pt.
- Minimum safe blood order (MSBO) can guide need for transfusion by the prior history of a surgeon performing the proposed elective procedure.

PREOPERATIVE PREPARATION
N/A

OPERATIVE PREPARATION
N/A

ANESTHESIA
N/A

WAKE UP AND EMERGENCE
N/A

ICU OR PACU

- Over half of ICU pts are anemic by lab criteria within 72 hrs of ICU admission.
- 1/7 ICU pts receive a transfusion per day.
- Over a third of all ICU pts receive a transfusion during their ICU course.
- Longer a pt stays in ICU, more transfusion therapy
- Transfusions are independently associated w/ increased length of ICU stay & increased morbidity & mortality.
- Use similar transfusion triggers for other settings, except tend to transfuse earlier if CNS or cardiac ischemia or infarction.

Indications for platelet transfusion

- Prevention/treatment of nonsurgical bleeding due to thrombocytopenia

- If possible, prior to transfusion, establish the reason for thrombocytopenia. When thrombocytopenia is caused by marrow failure, the following transfusion triggers are considered appropriate:
- If platelet count is <10,000 & no additional abnormalities exist
- If platelet count is 10,000–20,000 & coagulation abnormalities exist or there are extensive petechiae or ecchymoses
- If pts is bleeding at sites other than skin & platelet count is <40–50,000
- Pts w/ accelerated platelet destruction w/ significant bleeding (eg, autoimmune thrombocytopenia or drug-induced thrombocytopenia)
- The endpoint should be cessation of bleeding, since an increment in platelet count is not likely to be achieved. Prophylactic transfusion is not indicated in these disorders.
- Prior to surgical & major invasive procedures when the platelet count is <50,000
- Do platelet count & coagulation studies prior to the transfusion to guide subsequent therapy. During surgery on pts w/ quantitative or qualitative platelet defects, evaluate the adequacy of hemostasis by assessing microvascular bleeding.

Pts w/ bleeding and/or urgent invasive procedures on warfarin therapy. Vitamin K will reverse the warfarin defect in about 12 hrs.

Do not transfuse plasma products for volume expansion, for prophylaxis following cardiopulmonary bypass or as a nutritional supplement.

VON WILLEBRAND'S DISEASE

KARL WILLMANN, MD, AND D. B. COURSIN, MD

SCREENING AND EVALUATION

- Hematology consult

- Labs to determine subtype of vWD, as this will guide therapy.
- Baseline coagulation studies, including PTT, PT, platelet count (these may be normal), vWf antigen & ristocetin cofactor activity

PREOPERATIVE PREPARATION

- Consult w/ hematologist.
- Treatment w/ desmopressin (DDAVP) 1 hr prior to surgery to stimulate vWf release & factor VIII (both 2- to 5-fold), which is indicated in type I & transiently effective in IIa. It is absolutely contraindicated in type IIb (induces thrombocytopenia) & is of no help in type III or IV.
- Treatment for type IIb & III requires replacement of factors from recombinant vWf, recombinant factor VIII that contains vWf, or factor VIII preparation, which also contain varying amounts of vWf. Cryoprecipitate can also be used. The nonrecombinant preparations put the pt at risk for virally transmitted diseases & are not first choices when recombinant therapy is available. Type IV requires platelet transfusion, as there is a defect in the binding site on platelets for vWf.
- Desmopressin is given as 0.3 ug/kg IV or 75 ug to each nostril. Maximal effect in 30 min, duration 6–8 hrs. May need to redose btwn 8–12 hrs, as these are the half-lives of vWf & factor VIII. There may be a decreased response to desmopressin w/ repeated dosing, as it takes time to replete the stores of vWf & factor VIII.
- Antifibrinolytics (aminocaproic acid, tranexamic acid) may be helpful adjuncts for decreased destruction of fibrin clot & decrease excessive hemorrhage.
- Regional anesthesia is relatively contraindicated.
- Avoid antiplatelet drugs.

OPERATIVE PREPARATION

N/A

ANESTHESIA

- Induction
  - ➤ Use care w/ laryngoscopy.
  - ➤ Avoid nasal intubation.
- Maintenance
  - ➤ No special concerns
- If bleeding despite preparation & DDAVP, consider:
  - ➤ Virus-inactivated factor VIII concentrates
  - ➤ Cryoprecipitate (has vWF but carries infectious risk)
- Avoid antiplatelet drugs.

WAKE UP AND EMERGENCE

- Coughing w/ emergence & oral/tracheal suctioning may cause trauma & bleeding.

ICU OR PACU

- Continued monitoring of hemostasis & coagulation status. May need continued therapy for vWD.